Praise for *Making the Most of Bed Rest*

"It is my pleasure to endorse this honest and inspirational book about bed rest. In my eighteen years of practicing obstetrics and gynecology, I have taken care of many high-risk pregnancies. Women are pushing the envelope by getting pregnant older, having more twins, and also working more than in the past. Despite the many advances in medicine, we still rely on bed rest as the cornerstone for treating preterm labor, premature rupture of membranes, and hypertension. For the majority of women who are always juggling many things at once, bed rest can be extremely dispiriting. Support from family, friends, employers, and the medical system is crucial. This book will serve as a guide to help patients make the most of their 'time off.' Bed rest should be seen as an opportunity for self-reflection, quieting the mind, and finding strength from within, not as a punishment. Thank you, Barbara, for your inspiration."

—Leslie Kardos, MD, Chief of Gynecology,
and Director of Gynecologic Robotic Surgery
at the California Pacific Medical Center

"WOW! Congratulations to the author and also to her audience for being focused on the possibilities for healing! Bed rest—short- or longterm—is the process of adapting and healing. This book encourages both the patient and his/ her support system to gain an adaptive attitude and be open to 'adventure' in every part of life, including times of unexpected physical confinement. Bed rest then becomes the right method, and a gift, to help cure medical challenges."

—Craig N. Bash, MD, MBA, Neuro-Radiologist
and Associate Professor, Uniformed Services School of Medicine

"Now you can rest assured! Everyone experiences seasons in life when rest is required for healing—pregnancy, surgery, injury, recovery from illness—and this book brings a hopeful, positive perspective to those times. Peterson presents superb solutions for weathering new life conditions, and teaches us to utilize the opportunity for great productivity, and happiness. A must-read with every prescription of bed rest."

—Ame Mahler Beanland, coauthor of the *New York Times* best seller
Nesting: It's a Chick Thing and *Postcards from the Bump: A Chick's Guide to
Getting to Know the Baby in Your Belly*

"I have been active all my life and I know I would cherish this book if I ever required bed rest! I would want everyone in my support system to have a copy so there would be no roadblocks to finding new outlets for someone who has always relied on fitness. As a busy mother, I turn to my workouts to resolve every kind of stress. Should something unexpected occur, this book would be my personal guide to getting through what is, in truth, always possible: downtime!"

—Kara Douglass Thom,
coauthor of *Hot (Sweaty) Mamas: Five Secrets to Life as a Fit Mom*

"This is a book that none of us expect to need, but when recovery means little or no movement, there is no better resource! Most of us wouldn't see the silver lining that Peterson suggests for a naturally challenging and often unthinkable situation: bed rest. The book is a gift, and her positive attitude a blessing!"

—Maureen Roben, number-one American marathoner in 1987,
inducted to the Colorado Running Hall of Fame in 2009,
trainer of marathoners, and now a mother of two

"Barbara Edelston Peterson took seemingly negative situations—bed rest for a high-risk pregnancy in one instance, and being confined to a wheelchair due to injury in another—and made the most of them by not only coping, but thriving. As someone who's often sidelined from the sports I love due to various injuries, I believe Peterson's creative approach and positive attitude are spot-on. It's important to realize that our sports, or whatever we're used to doing as a healthy, mobile person, don't define us. And that given a large amount of time unable to move like we want to, can actually help us discover parts of ourselves that would have gone unknown, because we would never have made time for it otherwise. Peterson's guide is a must-read for survival, should anyone find themselves in a similar situation. She encourages us to not only cope, but to seize the day and thrive, be a whole person, even when confined to a bed or wheelchair."

—Lisa Jhung, contributor to *Runner's World*,
manager of runnersworld.com/trail, journalist, freelance writer and editor

"In *Making the Most of Bed Rest,* Barbara Edelston Peterson—the most energetic person I know—shares her experiences with courage and fortitude, then shows the rest of us how to be productive, empowered, and even grateful while recovering from physical confinement. A heartfelt thank you for initiating this positive path to wellness."

—Nina Lesowitz, coauthor of *The Courage Companion,*
and the bestseller *Living Life as a Thank You*

"I don't want to be defined as just an 'athlete.' Yet sport has become my north, my reason for structure. Removing that backbone from my day as with a 2012 bike crash, surgery and downtime, left me very disoriented. Barbara's practical advice will serve well any active athlete or individual. Bed rest sure can be an enriching time, for both body and soul."

—Dan Hugo, world-class professional triathlete

"Any time there is a special guide to help navigate through something totally foreign, such as bed rest, it really helps! Just knowing that others have gone through something similar aids in feeling less isolated. Barbara's book has it all, while being upbeat, ambitious, creative, and life-instructive. It focuses first on recovery and improved wellness, and then the ocean of opportunity to discover parts of life that would otherwise never be realized. A big bonus in every chapter is guidance for others involved in the bed rest experience, such as partners, children, parents, friends, the medical team, and hired help. Bed rest is not about being stuck or frustrated, rather it is a call to action in making the most of personal well-being while in recovery."

—Jamie Whitmore, motivational speaker,
XTERRA World Champion, cancer survivor, mother of twins

"This is a book that none of us expect to need, but when recovery means little or no movement, there is no better resource! Most of us wouldn't see the silver lining that Peterson suggests for a naturally challenging and often unthinkable situation: bed rest. The book is a gift, and her positive attitude a blessing!"

—Maureen Roben, number-one American marathoner in 1987,
inducted to the Colorado Running Hall of Fame in 2009,
trainer of marathoners, and now a mother of two

"As a world champion athlete, inspiring sports psychologist, and mother of successful and accomplished daughters, author Barbara Edelston Peterson illuminates every page of *Making the Most of Bed Rest* with care, love, wisdom, and positive focus. Whether challenged by a devastating injury or facing months of bed rest while pregnant, Barbara keeps her light high and bright by sharing this treasure trove of hope, inspiration, and practical advice for others faced with physical restrictions and life-challenging circumstances. Her book will inspire you to fully embrace the new life that will greet you beyond your bed rest days."

—Margie Lapanja, author of *The Goddess' Guide to Love*
and cookbooks, including *Romancing the Stove* and *Food Men Love*

MAKING
THE
MOST
OF
BED REST

MAKING THE MOST OF BED REST

TIPS, TOOLS AND RESOURCES FOR A REWARDING RECOVERY FROM ANY HEALTH CHALLENGE

BARBARA EDELSTON PETERSON

PREFACE BY DR. HALLIE BEACHAM

FOREWORD BY DR. CHRISTOPHER SEGLER

VIVA
EDITIONS

Published in the United States by Cleis Press, Inc.,
2246 Sixth Street, Berkeley, California 94710.

Printed in the United States.
Cover design: Scott Idleman/Blink
Cover photograph: Dougal Waters/Getty Images
Text design: Frank Wiedemann
First Edition.
10 9 8 7 6 5 4 3 2 1

Trade paper ISBN: 978-1-936740-16-1
E-book ISBN: 978-1-936740-37-6

Library of Congress Cataloging-in-Publication Data

Peterson, Barbara Edelston.
 Making the most of bed rest / Barbara Edelston Peterson. -- 1st ed.
      p. cm.
 Includes bibliographical references and index.
 ISBN 978-1-936740-16-1 (pbk. : alk. paper)
 1. Bed rest--Psychological aspects. 2. Pregnancy--Complications--Prevention. 3. Exercise. 4. Adjustment (Psychology) I. Title.
 RG572.P393 2012
 618.2'4--dc23
                                2012028810

To Hilary and Foreste, my daughters,
who have energized me to reach for the stars.
Thank you for your love and wisdom.

TABLE OF CONTENTS

xiii **ACKNOWLEDGMENTS**

xv **PREFACE** *by Dr. Hallie Beacham*

xvii **FOREWORD** *by Dr. Christopher Segler*

xix **INTRODUCTION**

1 **CHAPTER ONE** Finding Inspiration

9 **CHAPTER TWO** Immediate Preparation

17 **CHAPTER THREE** It's All About the Base Camp

27 **CHAPTER FOUR** Creating a Routine

31 **CHAPTER FIVE** The Power of Exercise

37 **CHAPTER SIX** Picnics in Bed

59 **CHAPTER SEVEN** Technology and Being Connected: A Guide to
Social Media Networks

73 **CHAPTER EIGHT** Personal Projects

89 **CHAPTER NINE** You're Not Alone

121 **CHAPTER TEN** Affection, Sexuality, and Bed Rest

127 **APPENDIX A** Positive Affirmations and Habits

131 **APPENDIX B** Personal Calendar and Journal

133 **APPENDIX C** Medical Team

137 **APPENDIX D** Postcards from the Bed

141 **APPENDIX E** New People and Resources

143 **APPENDIX F** Shopping Guide

147 **ABOUT THE AUTHOR**

ACKNOWLEDGMENTS

To my family: Dick, Hilary, and Foreste. Thank you for helping me to survive and thrive while enduring bed rest. Yes, I was out of my element for a long time, but we made it, *all of us made it with flying colors*! Thank you for the dedication not only to me, but also to the medical and spiritual components that fortified a complete recovery in both of my bed rest experiences. My writing this book took a whole other level of focus, patience, support, and faith in me. From my core, thank you! We did it all.

A sincere thank you to the following people for their love and support during bed rest number one in 1998: Dick, my husband; my mother and father, Joan and Gil; my sisters, Jeri and Jill; my niece Emily; Dee and Carrell; my doctor and friend Dr. Hallie Beacham; and family best friends, Ursula and Volker Flache. Thank you, Hilary, for ultimately cooperating within the womb, for staying two weeks past your due date, which allowed me to regain much needed physical strength. You emerged as a living angel, and you are still that beautiful individual at age twenty-two.

The following people reached out and provided unforgettable support during bed rest number two in 2010: Dick, Hilary, and Foreste, my immediate family; Jennifer Chapman, Erin Collum, Jack Bieda, Pam Johann, Jane Barrett, Ursula Flache, Steve Brown, Geri Charnin, Kevin Faulkner, Barry and Carolina Gustin, Margie Lapanja, and the staff and my friends at the Claremont, especially Shawel, Iasu, Mani, Marilyn, and Nellie. A special note in loving memory of our dog, Posie, whose unimposing and gentle nature helped me, and she shall never be forgotten. Foreste and Hilary, my dear ones, thank you for taking me on walks in the wheelchair, for driving and doing the necessary errands, for sharing your uplifting music and laughter, and for concocting extraordinarily delicious lunches and taking the time to eat together outside and picnic-style. Kindness is healing.

I am most indebted to Dr. Christopher Segler for his extraordinary brilliance and positive medical approach while working closely with me throughout the five-month process to complete recovery.

I am deeply appreciative of the many testimonial writers whose experiences are woven into the book's text.

Brenda Knight, and Nancy Fish, thank you for opening the doors at Viva Editions, and for helping provide this important resource not only for patients, but for medical teams and caregivers. Kara Wuest, your input made this book more worthy, and I cannot thank you enough for your steadfast efforts. Kitty Stryker, thank you for your contributions. Hera, your stunning aesthetics and overall clarity helped make this book possible.

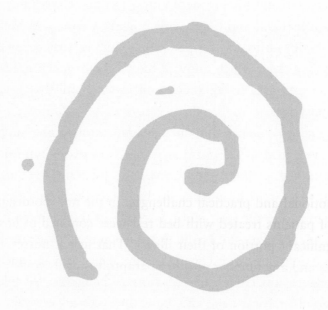

PREFACE

By Hallie Beacham, M.D., M.P.H.

Every year, legions of patients are prescribed bed rest as part of a treatment regimen. Many of these prescriptions are for obstetrical patients, orthopedic patients, accident victims, and ophthalmic patients. When prescribed for these persons, bed rest becomes as important as any potion or pill.

Bed rest, however, is more intangible than medication, and is invariably prescribed for a patient who is least apt to find this form of therapy welcome news. This is especially true for the pregnant patient who is being treated for preterm labor or the athlete who has broken both heels in a fall and cannot conduct normal functions due to non-weight-bearing restrictions.

As a physician, I routinely describe to patients the potential side effects of medications. I indicate how often the medications should be taken, and this information is reinforced by the pharmacist, who provides labels highlighting the most significant side effects. As an obstetrician, when I first began to prescribe bed rest as a part of a regimen to control preterm labor or other pregnancy complications, it seemed so simple and straightforward. Medical side effects might be blood clots in the legs, as a result of prolonged inactivity of the legs and the resultant decrease in blood flow; constipation could be an issue. What I did not initially anticipate were some of the other consequences of prescribing bed rest, such as the emotional and practical challenges. In the not-too-distant past, the vast majority of patients treated with bed rest were confined to hospitals for a much more significant portion of their illness. That meant nurses and occupational therapists and any number of other paraprofessionals could observe possible physical and psychological problems the patient developed, and minister to them.

Now, with patients spending far less time in hospitals and families dependent on two incomes, the fallout from the bed rest prescription frequently rests squarely on the shoulders of the "infirm"! For obstetrical patients, inactivity is frequently thrust on an unwilling recipient who is excited about her pregnancy but who has just been informed of an immense disruption in her life. She's frightened about the possible outcome of her pregnancy. At this time the mother often isn't considering her own comfort but rather the medical threat to her baby, and, as a result, she doesn't ask or retain important information about her prescribed bed rest. Being at home—not in a hospital where she might seek continual paraprofessional input—has added to the problems experienced by bed rest patients.

I began to learn of these concerns as patients returned for their visits and shared their experiences with me. Patients told me they were now working *only* four hours a day, not eight, or they were home but they were using the stairs seven times a day. Since then, I've learned to be very specific in defining "bed rest." The written word is an invaluable adjunct to instruction given in the office.

Having experienced bed rest for herself, Barbara Edelston Peterson found she wanted solutions to myriad issues presented by her confinement. As a result, she's produced a comprehensive guide to give the new bed rest patient and their caregivers a way to negotiate this experience in the most tolerable fashion possible. In this book, she also shares her lessons and invaluable words for medical professionals, caregivers, and friends of the patient prescribed bed rest.

By *Christopher Segler, D.P.M.*

As a foot and ankle surgeon specializing in the treatment of athletes, I have witnessed many struggles with the concept of rest, with bed rest, of course, being the most difficult to swallow. The interesting paradox is that those most resistant to bed rest (high-achieving professionals, "super" moms, and athletes) are the very ones who actually need it the most once it is prescribed. Whether a working mom juggling responsibilities, a busy professional, or a world-class athlete, no one with a full life wants to rest.

The day I met Barbara Peterson was one day I won't forget. I had heard of her. I knew she was a multiple world-champion triathlete. And there she was sitting in a wheelchair in her kitchen, instead of defending her European title at XTERRA Switzerland. She shrugged and said, "At least I'll get the chance to catch up on this book I've been writing." True rest does not come easy for a world champion.

I too have personally been forced to rest. I have also paid the price of not resting. I had a heat stroke while racing motorcycles. I had pneumonia during my surgical residency. I even had a stroke after knee surgery. I had pneumonia again after Ironman Florida one year. That time I started the race with a cold and set a new personal record, it nearly killed me. All of these rather unpleasant events were preceded by a common circumstance—lack of adequate rest. All were also followed by a common event—forced (and unwelcomed) rest.

My view of bed rest is twofold. I have suffered the consequences of physically working myself to the brink, and, as a physician, I try on a nearly daily basis to help others avoid the same predictable, preventable malady. But for those who have been advised that bed rest will help, I will concede that it is no easy task to comply.

This book will teach you why and how you can survive and thrive through your unwanted period of rest. You may resist it, you may not love it, but if you accept it, this critical time can and will serve you well.

You have made a brilliant choice in purchasing this book. Barbara knows of what she speaks. She is an accomplished author, entrepreneur, world champion triathlete, and wildly successful wife and mother. She lives the advice she would offer others. She has succeeded through hard work. And she has succeeded in resting when it mattered most.

The day I met Barbara she had a life-altering type of injury. Frankly it was questionable whether or not Barbara would ever run again. But today I have a message on my phone from her. I have not deleted it, and every twenty-one days I listen to it and then save it again. In that message she is calling after her first post-injury race: XTERRA West Championships. In her characteristic understated tone, she says, "Well, it wasn't pretty, but I won."

It is remarkable what patience and rest can achieve.

Christopher Segler, D.P.M., is America's "Doc on the Run," a ten-time Ironman finisher, and an award-winning foot and ankle surgeon.

INTRODUCTION

Making the Most of Bed Rest is a comprehensive handbook offering inspirational and practical guidance for those who are physically confined due to a temporary medical issue. In search of a way to make the most of my own bed rest experiences—first with a pregnancy complication and twenty years later with bilateral heel fractures—I learned many important lessons and discovered profoundly positive opportunities. Bed rest can be the "time of your life" when you and your support system (family, medical team, friends, and professional care providers) embrace the necessities and possibilities.

In early 1998, I was prescribed bed rest for three months due to preterm labor. With dedicated help from my husband, we pioneered our way out of feeling confined, while I remained in bed for one hundred days. By being open, innovative, and careful, the time was well spent albeit with its moments of natural frustration and discomfort. While lying flat or on my side the entire time, except to go to the bathroom, I sustained a healthy, spiritually fulfilling, and productive experience. Again, in 2010, as a mother of teenage daughters with an active career as a psychologist, author, and motivational speaker, and a "side career" as a pro triathlete traveling worldwide to compete, I found myself in a wheelchair for four months, after falling from high in my closet. While this experience offered more mobility than lying on my side with no detours between the bed and the bathroom, the process of healing fragile bones was sensitive and painstakingly slow. At the time of each medical emergency, I needed something that did not exist: a resource explaining how to best survive and even thrive in such restrictive conditions. I needed inspiration and specific direction and instructions on how to function in my new reality. Equally in need of guidance were my husband, our children, and the rest of my bed rest community.

There are millions of bedridden patients and others related to this predicament that can thrive, with simple instructions and enthusiastic suggestions, in the midst of immobility. Bed rest can be a positive and productive experience, as was my first bed rest experience where I "covered a lot of territory" while lying in one place. I "moved" into many exciting areas of life: I learned a language, explored film, immersed myself in various art projects, fulfilled personal and professional obligations, and enjoyed family and friends. I made a choice to endure this situation as best as I could, and while alone each day I used the time to my advantage. You can too!

I began my first bed rest journey by first shifting all of my expectations to one important goal: sustaining a healthy pregnancy. I learned a lot about my medical complications, and then I comfortably moved beyond them. With the second bed rest experience, I learned all I could about the calcaneus heel bone, and found courage quickly to pursue as normal a life as I could from the wheelchair. Each time on bed rest, I survived and thrived on an all-new daily timetable, and accepted that physical freedom was out of my control. This book carefully outlines the possibilities for a productive life on bed rest, and guides you, your family, and everyone in your circle of care (including the medical team) to stay positive and "active" while adhering to your medical needs. Throughout each chapter, you will find practical resources, emotional wisdom, creative ideas, and spiritual encouragement. And you will discover that in your state of immobility—whether you are bedridden due to a pregnancy complication, or recovering from an ophthalmic or orthopedic injury, or something as extreme as an organ transplant—there are ways to make the most of this unique and temporary time. Why not be energized and even renewed while you are safely quiet, promoting good health?

I encourage you to read through the pages, to find solace in the best approach for your individual circumstance. Please keep in mind this book is not medical or technical in nature. Reorienting and rechanneling your personal energy now and throughout the time on bed rest is key to a meaningful experience. Embracing the conditions and your environment will help you to move forward, prepare, and adapt. I am confident that you will discover options for coping, functioning, and feeling content.

Perspective. Faced with the initially shocking reality of bed rest, people often feel desperate, sad and stressed, scared and isolated. Loss of physical mobility presents unprecedented emotions and immediate lifestyle challenges. When you find yourself confined to a bed, couch, or wheelchair, it's only natural to feel distraught and even helpless. But your situation is temporary, not permanent. You have been given a medical prescription so that you optimally heal and recover. Do not lose sight of the fact that there is "light at the end of the tunnel." And there are plenty of ways to make the most of this new reality. I did it twice, and I not only survived the many hours and days of bed rest, I thrived on redirecting my energy to new and meaningful activities and taking advantage of the sanctuary of stillness.

Wired. Fortunately, we live in an era of advanced technology, and the bed rest experience is not as limiting as it was two decades ago when I was bedridden due to pre-term labor. Now, there are laptops, cell phones, satellite television, and wireless Internet providing a full range of opportunities for communication and entertainment. Social, professional, and medical networks are available wherever you are—at home or in the hospital.

Personal background. This kind of resource would have been invaluable to me when I was prescribed bed rest in the winter of 1989. There was nothing available offering practical guidance, and definitely nothing that offered compassion specific to the bed rest conditions, either at the doctor's office or in any book-store large or small (my husband checked every type of bookstore from hospital to boutique, to special university medical and psychology bookstores, to mega-bookstores like Barnes & Noble). Since we had no warning or adjustment period, which is most often the case for a bed rest patient, we looked to our doctor and her team for help, but they were too busy to provide much of anything except during my scheduled visits. We were on our own with little choice but to become bed rest pioneers. And so, through trial and error, we groped our way home from the hospital and the inventions began, and continued, throughout our journey. Unfortunately, we struggled, but we felt strong: "Where there's a will, there's a way!" We found our way tool by tool, accessory by accessory. A comfortable bed was paramount. Other practical problems multiplied, and so did our solutions. We had picnics in bed, and when I was left alone for most of the day, sometimes for twelve hours at a time, I had enough drinking water and food on or next to the bed. We organized the many necessary supplies without burying me in bed. We rigged up a safe power strip so that my electronics were charged without the fear of blowing fuses. We figured out how I would self-manage the wonderful bedpan, and last but not least, we found ways to embrace the occasional overflow of emotions that rarely announced their arrival. We learned to eliminate unneces-sary stresses that disturbed not only my peace but also the healing process (stress is indeed unhealthy for acute medical conditions). We agreed upon a "zero toler-ance" policy for particular visitors and overly stimulating films. Simple solutions such as open windows for fresh air, and an abundance of humor when spirits needed a lift, went a long way throughout the many days of my confinement.

Why a book? Toward the end of my first term of bed rest, I knew that I would have to share my tale of success. I produced the first edition in 1998, *The Bed Rest Survival Guide*. As a result of the recent double heel fractures, and the subsequent bed rest in a more modern era, I had more to share. Regardless of increased access to the world via the Internet, smartphones, and wireless com-puters, the feelings of isolation, fear, and frustration from bed rest are as present as ever. As a mother and wife with a demanding career, I felt stuck. My identity crumbled, and the raw ramifications of immobilization depressed me.

I needed a bed rest companion—a book loaded with compassion and courage, practical tips, and reminders of how to reframe my attitude to be positive and productive.

Bottom line. Millions of people are bedridden or immobilized each year, and most everyone survives the inconvenience. You can be one of the many who thrives!

I deeply believe that your experience can be a gift. The ability to endure and learn from being physically confined will make you stronger, and wiser, and will serve you throughout life. When you reach the end of this significant time, I believe you will agree that your greatest lessons may not be from the highs in life, or from doing one special thing, but from recognizing your inner strength to face challenges and overcome obstacles.

I recommend that you read the first two chapters immediately. They provide exactly what you'll need for basic bed rest survival. Once you have adjusted and everyone begins to adapt to the new conditions, the other chapters will help you "live more!" I hope you'll find a level of comfort and ways to be "active" and happy. May this book become a special companion, one that provides you with an abundance of positive reinforcement for optimal healing and for your complete recovery.

I welcome you to my website, www.bedrestwellness.com, and to contact me directly at barbara@bedrestwellness.com.

CHAPTER ONE

FINDING INSPIRATION

Under normal circumstances when we're tired and need rest, the bed is seductively warm and peaceful. Most of us love our beds! But when a doctor instructs us to remain in bed for an undetermined period of time, the context quickly changes, and what was a haven now represents a type of prison sentence.

Similarly, our favorite chair or couch is a place we welcome, where we land for comfort and relaxation after a day of work or a workout. It's the place where we spend hours reading and studying, watching a film, or talking with family and friends. None of us would volunteer spending days, weeks, and months in this same place, but sometimes to cure a temporary medical problem, we must.

At thirty-three years old and twenty-four weeks gestation with my first pregnancy, I went into preterm labor and was unexpectedly prescribed bed rest. At the time, the concept was foreign to me; I knew nothing about bed rest and its impact on lifestyle or how it would affect my sense of balance in my body, mind, and spirit. During the first moments of being told by my doctor that for the next three months I would have to stay very still in bed, I felt enriched by her special care, and spoke clearly in return, "I can do that." Dr. Beacham then explained that if the medical problems persisted, I would return to the hospital for the remainder of my pregnancy for monitored bed rest. I shook my head in obedience, and with a special type courage spoke three words, "whatever it takes."

My world then changed. I was hit with a shocking new reality, and my idea of a good life suddenly shifted. I wanted more than anything to stay at home in my own bed to "do" bed rest. Shaking in fear and disbelief that this was happening to me, I determined to do everything I could to secure my precious prenatal health and sanity. This was a first-time real life survival test.

Fast-forward twenty-two years. I heard the same instructions from an emergency room doctor just after falling from high inside my closet and breaking both heels. Now, as the mother of a mature family with a busy career as a writer and sports psychologist, and training incessantly as a triathlete, my world changed once again. Another term of bed rest with slightly more flexibility—the use of a wheelchair—was before me. That morning in the emergency room I shook my head once again, and in response to the attending nurse and doctor, I stated, "Yes, I understand immobility." But when they stepped away, my heart sank, the tears flowed, and my whole identity crumbled into many tiny pieces. Shaking in sadness this time, I turned inward, reflecting upon the courage I needed to endure bed rest number one. I would summon my creative and positive spirit. There were so many unfinished writing projects in my current life; I now had time to finish all of them! And this time, modern technology would make this bed rest experience much less isolating. I quickly found resolve to once again make the most of a very difficult situation. Life has its ways of teaching important lessons, often at just the right moment.

There are as many reactions to such an extreme change in lifestyle as there are approaches to enduring it. You are being forced to adapt to a radical change of lifestyle due to unexpected trauma beyond your control. Your initial reaction may be to feel trapped, distressed, and anxious. There may be a hurricane of emotions, and I encourage you to honor every feeling; there is reason to be shocked and overwhelmed. But move forward soon with strength and focus on making the most of bed rest. In being resourceful, you will become happy, productive, and healthy. Discover joy in the opportunities that will open to you.

Bed rest is not living death! It is a temporary way of life that has the potential to become an extraordinary experience because you and your support team can create a positive journey. The benefits will flourish when you embrace your situation fully: learn as much as you can about your medical condition, shift your attitude so that you begin to make the most of the experience, and align your entire support system with an open, innovative, and positive orientation. When you settle into bed, a couch, or a wheelchair, your thoughts naturally begin to reframe themselves (human nature: fight or flight) and you will naturally begin to mentally reorganize your new existence. While doing so, ask yourself the following questions for the sake of clarity, and if it helps, write out your answers: Who will I see during this time on bed rest? What can I do during the day? What must I do each day (morning, midday, evening)? How will I spend my time attending to medical and personal needs? How will I track my recovery—beginning, middle and end? Share this information with your caregivers (family, friends, professional care providers). Discuss your new medical priorities and personal expectations. Review the possibilities, and request that the biggest help anyone can provide is to be respectful and reinforcing. By going through these steps, you are establishing optimal parameters for healing, a supportive climate for surviving and thriving on bed rest. No one in the caregiver role can do his or her job well without input from you. Therefore, communicate your plan, your thoughts, and everything else you feel others should know! Over time, given that your physical and emotional conditions will change, a reevaluation and updated communication is imperative. Bed rest is a very special circumstance and while everyone has the best of intentions to help, it requires an abundance of patience, personal fortitude, and positive thinking.

Everyone who reads this book must keep in mind that every bed rest case is unique, and that what is practical, creative, and sensitive to one individual may be different to another. While there are countless reasons for bed rest, there are also huge variables in resources and recovery environments. Make it great!

With my first bed rest experience, before there were wireless technology, cell phones and laptops, it took several days to assess what would be needed and what was available so that I could function in a basic way. It was a major challenge to organize an effective way to communicate with key people, and coordinate systems to support a way to continue at my job. When this was all figured out, I began to thrive while staying in one place—my bed. For three months I stayed active *and* quiet. With the second bed rest, when I broke my heels, I was more mobile, moving from room to room via crawling or the wheelchair. Yet there were the initial tasks of organization and coordination so that I could optimally function. Then I was energized to focus on what I could do, not what I couldn't do.

The emotional landscape for every bed rest patient is initially rugged because there is little escape from the harsh reality of immobility. Yet, when life stabilizes, inner peace emerges along with a new level of inner strength. After the first week of bed rest—in both of my cases—the sharpness of fear and disappointment dissipated, and I accepted the change in my life.

I encourage you to be mindful of the roller coaster of positive and negative thoughts and behaviors. Look forward and be positive, as positive thoughts manifest into positive words, which become positive actions, and eventually positive habits. I never cursed my bed while on bed rest. Rather, I blessed it, as I was safe and in the right position for a healthy and full-term pregnancy. I never cursed the wheelchair, as it was the only vehicle that allowed me to be mobile while protecting my heels. In each case, I found a new kind of happiness. There is a way for you to find this, too.

The Journey Begins with Acceptance

The first way to create an optimal healing environment is through acceptance of your new bed rest reality. With acceptance, you will create the right type of conditions, and your focus and strength will turn to successfully enduring this epic life adventure. You have a choice to respond to this extraordinary medical prescription by lamenting it or by accepting it. I pondered over the famous serenity prayer that I had not understood as well as I do now, "God grant me the serenity to accept the things I cannot change, the courage to change the things I can, and the wisdom to know the difference." With acceptance, the emotional conundrum of being physically confined quickly dissolves. Once I accepted my new reality, I no longer felt lost, aimless, or worthless. Instead, I felt comfortable. New energy emerged along with a desire to be happy and productive.

In a survey of hundreds of people who experienced bed rest for various physical ailments, the majority agreed that with knowledge of the medical problem, the acceptance rate skyrocketed and the psychological burden of prolonged immobility subsided. In most cases, the patients' understanding of anatomical details prompted a higher degree of self-care, compassion and less protest of the bed rest prescription. Beyond acceptance and patience, for ninety percent of immobilized patients interviewed after their bed rest experience, it was an extraordinary and memorable experience, even life changing in a positive way. Whether a pregnancy complication, foot or ankle problem, back injury, degenerative hip, viral disability, or another medical condition that requires bed rest, this particular remedy is a small price to pay for the return to good health.

With acceptance and knowledge of the facts that are causing your medical limitations, you and your support team will better champion the days and weeks of bed rest. Being informed also ensures that helping hands (caregivers) are aligned with your medical matters. For example, in the early weeks of my first bed rest experience, none of my family, friends, or caregiver(s) grasped the severity of my situation. I simply could not—and did not—*get out of bed* or the contractions would resume with the possibility of a premature birth. Complete understanding and communication of specific medical details eliminates misconceptions and potential problems. Again, once you accept your situation, you can begin focusing on what you can do rather than what you cannot do. Charles Darwin said it best, "A man who dares waste one hour of life, has not discovered the value of life." Whether it be fulfilling your work from home, mothering your children from the bed, spending your days learning a new language, becoming financially literate, passionately reading every body of work by one author, lifting weights to build up your core while the injured part of the body remains still (with doctor's permission), or finishing the family photo albums, the opportunities abound. Loved ones and caregivers must fully understand the medical parameters in being responsible and positive players in the bed rest experience. Bed rest calls for acceptance of the present—good or bad. It provides valuable perspective, and new opportunities to be enriched with grace and wisdom.

Bed Rest as Teacher

In our culture, illness and physical disabilities are often viewed as problems that occur from outside us. Any inconvenience in the healing process is usually facilitated by the use of medication. Rarely are patients forced to endure stillness to heal or recover from their condition. What I learned by adapting to bed rest is that the process can be a marvelous teacher.

My bed rest experiences in 1998, and again in 2010, were defining moments, and two of the best life experiences I have ever had. From the beginning to the end of each episode, I grew profoundly as a person. In the face of adversity, my spirits moved from dark to light. Fear changed to self-confidence, and heavy doubt gave way to hope and empowerment. During the hours that I lay quietly in bed, I learned to depend on myself for problem solving and also for contentment. I discovered personal interests I never knew existed. A new world of ingenuity, experimentation, innovation rose from being horizontal! I felt strong and capable, using mental skills that later enriched motherhood and daily life. Challenges, large or small, offer opportunities to think and act differently.

Bed rest will show you that you possess the ability to change your life when you need to—to travel a new road and not feel lost. Whether on bed rest, in a wheelchair, swimming the deep seas, or climbing to the top of a mountain, you are the driver, and the healer is within.

An old Chinese saying inspired me to stay positive, to see the hours before me as golden, and to use my time wisely: "An inch of time is an inch of gold: Treasure it. Appreciate its fleeting nature; misplaced gold is easily found, misspent time is lost forever."

Being bedridden at the young age of thirty-three years old, encouraged me to look at the patterns throughout my life, and see that setbacks are inevitable, and that life is an ever-changing process. I learned firsthand that progress can happen slowly, and in small doses, and that in the midst of life's journey, accomplishment rises out of tenacity, patience, and a positive attitude.

I saw bed rest as a bump along the path of Life, a rough spot that can offer invaluable lessons. Norman Cousins, a scholar and journalist who devoted much of his time to the issues of illness and healing, wrote, "The greatest force in the human body is the natural drive of the body to heal itself—but that force is not independent of the belief system, which can translate expectations into physiological change. Nothing is more wondrous about the fifteen billion neurons in the human brain than their ability to convert thoughts, hopes, ideas, and attitudes into chemical substances. Everything begins, therefore, with belief. What we believe is the most powerful option of all."

CHAPTER TWO

IMMEDIATE PREPARATION

Humans are active energy systems in all conditions, but surprisingly so while coping with bed rest. There is much to manage for short- and long-term comfort and health. Your first priority is to focus on your immediate needs, such as the role of caregivers and how to develop new systems to effectively function while immobilized. The real "rest" will begin after the immediate preparation takes place.

Begin planning the following: communication for daily living; tools and other practical requirements for your comfort and optimal health; systems for the continuation of your family, career, and social involvements; and overall functionality of your bed rest existence.

You probably imagined that bed rest meant your whole world would stop, but it cannot, and will not! Once your support system is in place, and the necessary tools and accessories for eating, working, and living are coordinated for you then you will survive, if not thrive, on bed rest.

Please note: The following guidelines are generalized as bed rest conditions vary according to medical issues, the patient's home or hospital environment, extended care, and the patient's personality. Please use the suggestions in this book to your every advantage, and in accordance with your current medical, physical, and emotional capacity. Address any concerns or questions with your medical team. My hope is that you, your family members, friends, and care providers will quickly discover the best systems for your functioning and healing!

First Things First—The Essential Checklist

Call all of the important people in your life: family, colleagues, friends, and local community members (from your workplace, school, synagogue or church, book club, athletic friends, etc.) to let them know you are on bed rest or in a wheelchair in temporary physical confinement. You should not be isolated; you will need all the support and help you can get.

Arrange for access to your home. A key should be hidden somewhere outside or with a doorman so that only with your direction, select people can enter your bed rest environment. Expect to receive visitors and helpers; however, try to prevent a stream of steady traffic at least right away (visitors are wonderful but require energy that when out of balance is a distraction, takes away from happiness, and invites stress). Provide significant people with their own key(s); someone should make the extra keys for you to distribute wisely, keeping track of the names in list form. Everyone else shall receive instructions from you as to how to obtain a key and enter. Release this information wisely and communicate to each individual that access information is confidential (important, do not assume people automatically understand your need for privacy and security). You should personally schedule all of your visitors (keep a schedule in your phone or on the computer, in the scheduler in this book, or on a calendar by your bed). Be clear when you do not want someone to visit by stating directly when it is uncomfortable or inappropriate for a visit. Honor your new boundaries; it will reduce unnecessary stress. Example: After one visit from my boss, a wonderful person but very hyper, I had to request we continue to work over the telephone rather than face-to-face. His exuberance caused an increase in my contractions, absolutely counterproductive to healing. With my bilateral heel injury, a friend enthusiastically came to visit, and once here, took every phone call on her cell, began yelling at workmen at her home, and proceeded to call her husband screaming about the incompetent construction workers. There was enough stress from my injury, and there wasn't space for more. Important: Make sure the key is returned to its place each time!

Organize and document new contact information: doctors, nurses, care providers, neighbors, hospital help lines, physical therapists, etc. Edit as needed; keep in your cell phone or on paper by your bed. Fill out the form in Appendix E, your contact list of new people and resources.

Call your insurance carrier. You must be crystal clear about the facts of your medical situation. Inform your insurance of the injury, illness, or medical condition, explain that you will need home care, and inquire about what your insurance covers: home care assistance, bed and wheelchair rental, physical therapy and massage, miscellaneous medical supplies (special mattress, bedside toilet, able table, tools for reaching and picking up materials, book holders, reading lights). If you are pregnant, you may want to inquire about coverage in the event of complications during bed rest or delivery (cesarean section) or extra care if your baby is born prematurely. Inform yourself of pertinent bed rest coverage and other insurance issues. Knowing what is paid for, and what is possible to do while bedridden is a great source of comfort. My weekly massages were covered by insurance, and it made such a positive difference!

File for disability insurance. Call your local Employment Development Department and have the papers sent to your home, or review direct online services. Call your employer's Human Resources Manager/Director to obtain all necessary instructions for compensation during your absence. You may need your doctor's and/or employer's signature; if there is no printer in your home, be prepared to have all EDD and/or Human Resources hard copies mailed to you.

IMMEDIATE SUPPLIES
FOR IMMEDIATE COMFORT

Cell or cordless phone (with chargers and power outlet near bed)

Good mattress (purchase an egg crate mattress)

Supportive pillows

Bedside table

On-the-bed table or an "able table"

Small case for pens, pad of paper, glasses (reading or other Rx glasses)

Small cooler(s) to place on bed

Water bottle with larger supply of water nearby (two large bottles filled with water)

Laptop with wireless Internet connection

Lightweight cot for mobility to other parts of home or outdoors

Cash, as you will want to reimburse people who help with errands. Do not give just anyone a blank check or your ATM card.

Hired Help and Caregivers

Hire housekeeping assistance if you can afford it. Ideally, this person should have a car to do errands for you outside the home: banking, post office, grocery shopping, and anything else. Assistance inside your home may include meal preparation, laundry, and personal organization. Don't expect your partner to do everything as few people can work, clean, shop, attend to a loved one who is confined to a bed or wheelchair, take care of their own needs, and communicate to others who are inquiring as to the status of the patient!

Your "job" is to clarify your needs to all hired help, whether or not you are looking for household and/or medical assistance. Many caregivers provide a combination of services: light housekeeping, shopping, meal preparation, laundry, as well as helping with medical care and personal hygiene. Costs for such services vary, and there may be a minimum time requirement. You will probably want the same person each visit for the duration of bed rest. Shop around. Personal referrals are preferable. Always do a background check. Involve a family member, friend, or someone in your community for an extended job as your care provider, only under these conditions:

You are comfortable around the person, without inhibitions;

He or she is mature and sensitive to your unique set of circumstances, respects you, understands your need for quiet, private time, and supports your personal family relationships (without feeling left out); and

He or she demonstrates compassion, emotional stability, a positive demeanor, maturity, and is able to entertain oneself while waiting.

You can also organize care and get your needs met through a variety of online resources. Websites such as lotsahelpinghands.com, sharethecare.org, carecalendar.org, and mealbaby.com are useful tools to organize people around visiting you, bringing you supplies, and arranging food delivery. Someone else can also maintain these sites for you after you share what you would prefer in terms of timing and specific wishes. These sites work especially well when kept current and updated and can help let people know how you are doing.

Home Delivery Services

Become familiar with local delivery services in your neighborhood or surrounding region. When appropriate, explain your situation. Be prepared by having a well thought-out explanation of the situation, and expectations, i.e., does the delivery service use the hidden key, is it one and only one person who comes through the front door and/or into the bedroom, etc. Home delivery can include the following: grocery shopping; pharmacy visits; meal preparation (also see chapter 6, Picnics in Bed); transportation services for children; dog walkers; gardeners; and laundry and dry cleaning.

Answering the Repeated Question, "What Can I Do to Help?"

Part of your immediate preparation is having a plan to answer the question you will hear many times, from many people: "What can I do to help?"

You will need help from beginning to end of your time on bed rest. People like to help! A grateful and clear reply motivates others who want to reach out. Be ready with specifics (keep a list on your phone, bedside paper, or in a word document) and always express thanks! Important: always communicate your ability to reimburse for all purchases, or arrange for advanced payment.

Examples of responses: "Thank you for asking! There are a few things around the house that I would like to have closer to me, or that I would like to check on. I have a short list, and when you come over, would you mind helping with that?" or "Thank you for asking! Would you mind picking up Bill's dry cleaning on your way. I've got money here to pay you back. It would be a huge help!" or "Thank you for asking! It would be wonderful if you came for a short visit, and while you're here, would you mind watering the plants? That would be a big help today," or "Oh, I would love to have a visit, and as far as helping, it would be great! Would you mind emptying the dishwasher at some point while you're here? Every little bit makes a huge difference!" or "Oh, thank you for asking. You have such a beautiful garden. What I need more than anything today is a flower to look at! Would you mind bringing something special from your garden? When you get here I'll tell you where you can find a vase. This is what I need more than anything else today!" or "Oh, thanks for being concerned. More than anything I just need someone to watch a film with me. Do you have the time, and would you be interested? I can download a great one, and be all ready soon after you arrive."

Planning Your Needs

If you aren't sure what you'll need help with, here are some examples of bed rest patients' needs:

Picking up groceries. Have the shopping list ready or call ahead if you have a neighborhood grocery. Someone's "job" for you could be to take ownership of your grocery status, the supply and food inventory and the fulfillment when it is depleted. When you are managing medical issues and confined, the issue of maintaining your food supply takes on another level of importance; you never want your staples and fresh goods to get too low. When beginning the process of managing your foods while physically confined, explain your situation to a local grocery store, inquire with the manager if someone there can shop for the duration of your time on bed rest, while stating that a designated helper will pick it all up at a designated time. If you don't already have a charge account, check on the possibility of opening one. Otherwise, devise a special arrangement to pay for the shopping either with a credit card or providing one large payment to cover the purchases over a period of time. You can also order food and supplies online and have them delivered to your house. Make sure you get the help you need to unload and put them away.

Bringing in the mail.

Mailing personal correspondence, bills, packages, etc.

Picking out and purchasing gifts for family, friends, helpers on special occasions. Consider asking them to have the gift wrapped with a small blank card included (you can write on it once it's in your hands).

Shopping for home office supplies, stamps, art, and personal project supplies. Stamps can be purchased online or via mail order.

Child transportation. Having others picking up children is very sensitive, and you must secure this arrangement with the utmost of trust and confidence in the help. Try to create a routine schedule involving the same driver and destination(s). Make sure to communicate all the details to all parties involved, especially to children. Reducing stress is possible with telephone check-ins.

Given your level of immobility, each visit from someone can and should be combined with accomplishing an errand. Use the "Personal Calendar and Journal" in Appendix B as a guideline to help coordinate your helpers and the various tasks.

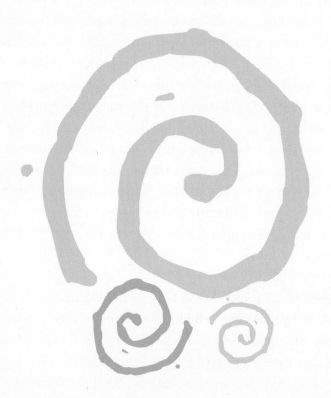

CHAPTER THREE

IT'S ALL ABOUT THE BASE CAMP

If you are bedridden, this chapter is your bible. If you are bound to a wheelchair or you are immobilized in another way, please use the guiding principles and creative suggestions where applicable.

Bed

Welcome to your new home base, known by millions of bed rest patients as "Command Central" or "Base Camp." The bed, the couch, the leather recliner—wherever you have settled to endure this time of stillness—becomes the base of all operations, the place that "holds" everything that you do. When this environment is comfortable and organized, it is functional and enjoyable. And while a change of scenery helps and I enthusiastically encourage changing resting locations when possible, it is from one main base that you will proceed forward over the next weeks and possibly months. From this setting, the many different aspects in your life will take place: healing, eating, sleeping, working, parenting, socializing, being creative, enjoying fitness (a little is better than none only per doctor's approval), and everything else.

The bed and immediate surroundings must be modified to function as your all-important foundation for short- and long-term wellbeing. You may want or need to relocate your bed; renting a hospital bed or buying a portable cot to position yourself more centrally in your home is a good option. You may choose to utilize different beds in several locations, for instance, putting a cot outside in the garden, one in the kitchen, and another in the children's playroom. Lowering your bed(s) close to the floor will enhance parenting young children. Or, if there is an injury involved such as a foot, knee, or hip injury, a low bed position will provide better options for your limited mobility. When children are involved while you are bedridden, a low bed provides greater ease and safety, and overall less stress when diapering or when little ones are climbing on and off the bed. Use of a waterbed requires approval from your doctor.

The Accessorized Bed

Creating an environment that is pleasant and comfortable (don't underestimate the value of this), and that supports being "active" and productive, is paramount to having a positive bed rest experience.

The following list of accessories will help you to attain an ideal environment. If these suggestions lead you and your caregivers to new ideas, go with it; now is the time to be innovative! Apply every available tool to elevate you far beyond the limits imposed by bed rest. Taking the time and making the effort to be comfortable and functional is minor in comparison to the benefits you will receive. Plan to share the load. Ask for help researching accessories, making phone calls, shopping for your needs, and the physical installation of a new bed. Your support team will be happy to help make your base great!

Healing begins on a mattress: egg-crate, medical air, and pressure reduction foam are all good choices. The mattress is the number-one priority as it plays a critical role in providing long-term comfort and support. Mattresses are designed to provide distinct physical support, so depending on your medical issue, there are various options. The right mattress reduces pressure on hips, knees, elbows, and one's overall body. Research the Internet for "medical mattress" or call medical supply stores, pharmacies, and foam mattress outlets to obtain important details including a survey of prices. When shopping, keep in mind that a new mattress with a strong plastic or synthetic odor may be unpleasant as well as unsafe (toxic or allergenic). Consider organic and hyper-allergenic products when choosing a new mattress. For this, search "natural organic mattress and bedding."

I discovered the egg-crate mattress with my first bed rest experience, and since that time, I have never been without this type of mattress, including one on each of my children's beds. Another option is the medical air mattress, which has a mechanism that allows you to customize the firmness for each side with the touch of a button.

Bed Accessories:

Bolster—A firm back pillow that supports your back if you must lie on your side. You can either buy one or make one by taping rolled blankets (four or five usually work).

Lamb's wool mattress pad—Helps keep the body warm in winter and cool in summer. It also has a great touch to the skin.

Several pillows, in different styles and sizes—A minimum of three extra pillows will provide immediate comfort during bed rest. Depending on your situation, you'll want to have more available for your legs, your back, and your side. Neck support pillows (egg-crate foam), body pillows, adjustable bed wedge, leg incliner are all therapeutic options for bedridden patients.

Temple pillow—A small, silk pillow for relaxing the head and forehead, it can even be precooled in the freezer or refrigerator.

"Nice" sheets—Sheets can make a positive difference for personal comfort and happiness. Flannel sheets in the winter are helpful for maximizing warmth and relaxation. Bright-colored sheets can help make your environment a little brighter. Bold prints hide food stains that are inevitable, and potentially annoying to see. Smooth satin sheets allow for easy turning in bed. Cotton sheets are refreshing, and over time, more comfortable to the touch than polyester sheets.

Blankets—Your level of warmth equals your level of relaxation, which translates into your ability to focus on healing, not working to stay warm. Polar fleece will provide warmth without the weight of a traditional wool blanket. Speak with your doctor about using an electric blanket. This may not be advisable for certain medical conditions, particularly pregnancy.

On-the-Bed Tools and Other Bed Rest Accessories:

Reading light(s)—You may be reading or writing at unusual hours, and it is important that you have plenty of light, while at the same time not bothering any one in the same room. Or, you may need to check your medicines numerous times throughout the night, or change a bandage, or time contractions if you have preterm labor, or write in a journal for your medical team, coaches, or yourself. A Petzl headlamp next to your bed, a flashlight on your cell phone, or a clamped-on bed light will help! They are all easily located at local camping stores, Barnes & Noble, Amazon.com, and Levenger.com.

Lap tray or "able table"—This is a lightweight table that rests on the bed, and becomes a personal workbench. It's a tool with multiple functions: eating tray, reading and writing surface, creative project table, and computer use. A six-position solid wood tray with laminate top for easy cleaning is recommended.

Over-bed table with wheels—This is a key multipurpose organizer. Ideally it is stationed next to the bed serving as the main holding surface for items that are used on a daily basis. It is designed to swing over the patient's lap for ease of reach and be pushed away when the items are not needed. A table with an adjustable height, made of wood with a stain-resistant top is highly recommended. Suggestion: if your table is on a carpet, you may want to try a plastic carpet protector to ensure mobility of the table's wheels.

The healing continues by keeping supplies, communication tools, and personal objects nearby and orderly, which increases energy for healing, productivity, and creativity.

For the Bedside Table:

    Sanitizing and general clean up hand-wipes

    Chapstick, lip gloss, hand cream

    Telephone (recommend cell or cordless with a headset for
        head and neck comfort)

    Laptop computer, earphones, headset

    Books

    iPod with mount and speakers

    Water bottle—hydration is your best friend

    Makeup bag with mirror

    Tissues

    Toothpicks

    All medications (label the tops and sides of every vial; always
        use childproof caps for the safety of your own or visiting
        children)

    TV remote control

    Clock

    Pens and pencils

    Paper, sticky notes, stationery

    Clipboard

    Stamps

Supply holder on bedside table—This reduces clutter while providing one point of access to pencils/pens, notepad, remote control, wallet/cash/credit cards, and any other small items. It also prevents temporary and frustrating losses. A rectangular plastic container, small bucket, or an artist's toolbox all work well for this.

Small cooler—This is particularly useful if you are alone for extended periods of time. It should contain healthful foods and drinks.

Reacher or picker-upper—Extends your reach by picking up or suctioning objects around the bed or on the floor.

Massage tools and foam roll—Therapeutic massage tools are compact, light, adjustable, and incredibly helpful for attending to aches and pains and tightness in the neck, buttocks, hips, and back. Search "massage tools" online for all options; fitness stores are an excellent local source.

Small fan—Air circulation is important for simulating wind and fresh air, and for enhancing healing and enriching energy for a positive and productive attitude. Note: Fifty percent of all illness is related to poor air circulation therefore a fan is helpful!

Bib—Eating may be messier than usual.

"Beyond" the Bed

A pleasant environment keeps the overall energy positive, and can be accomplished in many ways.

Bring the outdoors in!—Ideally, there is a window in your room, and maybe you've got a view. If so, regardless of the weather and climate, open the shades and window. Shower yourself and the bed with fresh air, sunshine, clouds, sounds, and smells from the outside world. I had an open window in my bedroom from February to May, where I lay very still to prevent preterm labor. When the weather turned cold, I wore a cap and down jacket, but the window stayed open! With fresh air came hope, and it helped me to feel enlivened when I might otherwise have felt lethargic and discouraged.

Gardening—Other uplifting elements are freshly potted plants and cut flowers in clear water. There is affirmation in their beauty, vibrant colors, sweet fragrance, and connection to nature. The process is so positive, and metaphoric for being open, patient, and willing to grow.

Surround the bed with photographs—Invite favorite people and places around the world into your room by surrounding the bed with photographs.

Be in beautiful company—yourself—Attractive robes, pajamas, or loose-fitting outfits will make you feel better, look better, and heal faster. This form of self-care is small but powerful. It's an effective boost to self-esteem, the backbone of strength, optimism, and wellness and an expression of pride, love, and generosity, inner brilliance and outer wellness. I wore fresh pajamas, colorful ribbons in my waist-long hair, and light makeup every day, for one hundred days. People who visited me said I looked vibrant, glowing and that I was a true inspiration. They saw the reflection of what I felt inside. During my second round of bed rest, mobile only by crawling or the wheelchair, I wrestled every morning trying to get into normal clothes. I applied the creams and makeup without a mirror, and onto my arms, I sprayed my favorite perfume. I dressed not for others, but for myself, so that each day I felt a sense of inner pride and love, fuel for healing and going far beyond the physical confinement of two broken heels. Messy hair, dry skin, a scruffy beard, old and tattered pajamas, and body odor is not motivating, for self or others.

Keep your mind stimulated—Having fun, feeling excitement, and thriving on all types of stimulation can help you transcend the deadness of immobility. Get out the iPod, Kindle, or laptop; download playlists, podcasts, films, and audiobooks. Turn up the volume, be engaged, laugh, gain wisdom, let the time pass. Certain times in the day are difficult; I used these periods for this type of entertainment. A word of caution: resist listening to or watching anything that increases your heart rate, i.e. films in the horror, psycho-thriller, violent genre or intensive music such as free-form jazz, heavy metal, or rap. Stress (of any type) is counterproductive to healing. Time spent peacefully and productively is the best way to make the most of your time on bed rest.

Stay connected—A cell phone is a multimedia device, a superb connection to the outside world, and the ideal security tool. If and when you change resting locations throughout the day, bring the cell phone; keep it close to you always. No need to feel overly detached or attached, as it is your time to be self-caring and selective about making and receiving calls. Your welfare is paramount while you are on bed rest. You are not obligated to normal daily processes, such as answering and responding to every incoming call. Simply keep the phone by your side, turn off the ringer while keeping on vibration, with no risk of missing important medical calls from your doctor or nurse, or being able to call out in the case of an unexpected disturbance or difficulty. Use of an earpiece (Bluetooth) or the phone's speaker feature offer options for more relaxing conversations, by easing your arm and neck, and using the technology to transmit your voice. Similarly, while working on the computer or on other projects with your hands, you can chat hands-free.

The power of social media—Multimedia health updates will take a load off your time and energy. Utilize the main social networks Twitter and Facebook, record a detailed voicemail report (replace your normal greeting), and write a weekly email to inform others of your medical and overall condition. This will greatly relieve having to repeat the information, eliminating unnecessary fatigue and stress.

Respect your environment—Reduce and/or eliminate clutter! When surfaces are free, you are free. Recycle or shelve magazines, newspapers, or books. I witnessed firsthand the overwhelming and negative effects of unkempt piles and clutter while interviewing bedridden patients. Invite a helper to purge your materials and to continually keep your spaces organized.

Remove garbage and waste—Don't let tissue, opened envelopes, mail, food wrappings, or unused bags collect near or around you. Once a day invite a helper to manage your area to keep the bed and surrounding areas free of waste. A clean environment reinforces clean thinking, positive emotions, and productive habits. You will feel more energized and heal more optimally in a neat environment.

Ensure privacy and comfort—Use a sound screen. It's a nifty mechanical device that filters noise. It can be used to capture unwanted background noise or to add noise if there is too much quiet in your surroundings.

Change your surroundings!—If you are able to change your bed locations by moving from your main bed to a couch, cot, or foam mattress, do it. From time to time, set up an alternative bed in the kitchen during mealtimes, or in the living room for visitors, or outdoors, if the weather permits. I loved talking with my husband while he cooked our dinners every evening; the cot barely fit in the small space, but we made it work. I also spent the majority of each day in our backyard, reading and working on my laptop in fresh air. The sun was therapy for relaxation and feeling positive. There are viable alternatives to lying in the same bed day after day: camp cot, inflatable raft, futon, couch, foam mattress, lounge chair, couch cushions, or plywood with pillows.

Bed rest is an opportunity to redirect personal energy and exercise personal will to make the most of whatever Life presents.

Bathroom Strategies

For some of you who are bedridden, the bedroom and the bathroom are one and the same. A bedpan or urinal replaces the toilet, and hair washing becomes a pastime. This is where acceptance gets exercised on another level, and a good laugh becomes as useful as a good cry! Do whatever you can to simply be a good sport while practicing all-out ingenuity. There is little argument that this degree of confinement is challenging.

When I was in this situation at the beginning of my heel injury, a friend came to visit, with the intent of helping me keep everything in perspective. Sure, everything felt out of my control due to not being able to bear my own weight but there were so many things I could do. A short while before, this friend broke both of her arms when she fell while running. Although it was not required that she lie still in bed, she was intensely restricted. She couldn't be left alone for six weeks, and her caregivers—her sister, her husband, and hired professionals—prepared her meals, fed her, bathed her, brushed her teeth, put in her tampons, and wiped her each time after she went to the bathroom. She explained to me with a wink, "Barb, this was just one of life's magical adventures!" Evidently, she found special ways to be patient and happy! Others with similar restrictions—women with complicated pregnancies who cannot move from the bed and who are also unable to use a normal toilet or wash their body or hair—find solace in portable shampoo basins, professional hairstylists, whole body hygienists, and masseurs who sponge bathe!

See the next page for bathroom safety considerations.

SAFETY FIRST

. . . .

If you are able to walk or wheelchair to a bathroom, the following items are worth considering for general assistance and increased security:

Safety bar in the tub and shower and by the toilet

Transfer bench for lowering into the tub

Bath seat for shower or sponge bath

Contoured toilet seat designed for comfort and security

Bath mats to prevent slips in bath or shower

Table and cup by the sink for medications or other health supplements you prefer to keep in the bathroom, e.g. vitamins, laxatives, pain relievers, or other health remedies.

Toothbrush and toothpaste should also be readily available.

Your time on bed rest is temporary. Take it as one of life's adventures.

CHAPTER FOUR

CREATING A ROUTINE

Bed rest and physical confinement is not the same for every patient. While millions of people a year are given this type of prescription to cure a temporary medical problem, there are varying conditions and requirements. Some people may be forced into a four-month rest to assure complete stabilization of internal organs or bone fractures, with permission only to use the bathroom. Others may be required to lie flat on their backs, or stomachs, unable to move at all. Many patients are not only confined to a bed, but also to the hospital where their medical condition is medically sensitive and close monitoring occurs multiple times a day. A select group of patients may be restricted from activity, but able to sit up on a couch or bed, or in a wheelchair. No matter what kind of bed rest has been prescribed, each day is important, and brings you closer to reaching your goal of resuming your normal lifestyle.

During the first days of bed rest, it is easy to feel like doing absolutely nothing other than lying on the bed, drifting in and out of sleep. Depending on your condition, you may also feel unsure of how to begin taking care of "business as usual." Eventually, you will reorient, yet without a compass for this sudden change of life, it is natural to feel hesitant about how best to proceed.

Creating a routine that is active and meaningful helps provide structure and purpose to each day. Within the first week, you will discover the ramifications of your condition, and you will understand what is possible to do and how the timing works best with family and caregivers. A new routine emerges naturally; however, holding on to your normal routine is not a bad thing to do. You will see that with a mix of obligations and activities, there is plenty to do each day, and that being restricted takes nothing away from being vital!

A routine and a daily schedule also serve to track progress, significant events, and milestones related to your medical condition. This type of information is significant and energizing; it helps to observe and embrace progress, all of which is emotionally gratifying and increasingly stabilizing.

The Daily Schedule

Many of you live by an organized schedule, which is the same thing as your daily routine. You probably keep a schedule in your cell phone or in a special book that includes appointments, meetings, deadlines, social engagements, and other events. Some of you may not be oriented this way; however, I suggest to everyone reading this book—the patient and the caregivers—that for this special time on bed rest, you keep a daily schedule that also tracks important medical events. Your old and new schedules can be merged but creating a brand new schedule for the many new facets of your current existence will become very helpful. This is a practical way to take charge of your unique situation, keeping a specific calendar and record of the daily activities involving the current medical obligations, contact information for the medical team, physical therapist(s), and care provider(s). Organizing your appointments, answering the inevitable questions pertaining to your condition on a specific day, making detailed observations and other medical concerns are all encouraged.

Keeping a daily schedule reinforces your active participation in your care and healing process. Reviewing your reality after the first few weeks you may want or need to change and improve how you spend your time including how you schedule appointments. A side benefit to keeping a daily schedule: you may have to explain to some people that you are too busy for a visit, and when you have a calendar in front of you, it's easier to say no with directness and a good conscience. A daily routine and schedule also assures that you are using your time in a meaningful, health-oriented, minimally stressful, and self-nurturing way.

Sample of my routine daily schedule:

7:00	Wake up
7:05	Begin the day with an Affirmation and review the Personal Calendar
7:15	Bathroom time, personal grooming
7:30	Breakfast and medications if applicable
8:00	Journal: Medical progress/personal monitoring
8:00–5:00	Drink water
9:00–Noon	Professional obligations: 2 to 4 hours
10:30–11:30	Fitness/physical therapy (see chapter 5)
10:30	Morning visitors/helpers
12:30	Lunch and medications if applicable
1:00	Personal grooming and affirmations
1:30–3:00	Professional obligations:1 to 2 hours
3:00–6:00	Afternoon visitors/helpers
4:00–6:00	Entertainment: film, reading, creative projects
6:00	Medical progress/personal monitoring
6:30	Dinner and medications if applicable
	Evening time with select people: partner, family, and friends
10:00	Sleep

Someday, you will look back on this time and say, how did I ever manage this? Your Personal Journal will be a type of scrapbook, and living proof that you not only did it, but that you did it well!

CHAPTER FIVE

THE POWER OF EXERCISE

Fitness and bed rest may seem like an oxymoron, but the right type of exercise is a tremendous benefit to most everyone who is physically confined. Only with prior doctor's approval, exercising certain parts of your body sustains some fitness, reduces atrophy, encourages blood circulation, elicits balance (less stress, better moods), and improves appetite and sleep patterns. Light exercise also helps relieve swelling and stiffness that frequently occurs from being physically limited over time.

Physical therapy and massage complement whatever forms of exercise are possible for you, and offer ways to help reduce pain or discomfort. Whatever "movement" you pursue during bed rest must be pre-authorized by a doctor, and all should be overseen by a physical therapist or certified home care specialist. Having someone else move and manipulate the body is common among bed rest or wheelchair patients.

While you are physically confined, any physical regime that you embark upon should be personalized. And once you begin, you must stay acutely aware of the impact on your body (no one else can feel what you feel). If at any time the exercises you are doing make you feel uncomfortable (in the case of pregnancy you feel increased contractions or in the case of a back or hip injury you feel increased pain), stop immediately. If you are taking medication that is known to increase your heart rate and cause shortness of breath, you need to be especially aware that your heart rate does not exceed 120 beats per minute at any time.

Light and limited exercise is powerful. It helps to prevent atrophy, and promotes mental clarity and spiritual vitality. Too much exercise, or the wrong kind of exercise, can cause serious problems such as infections, stress fatigue, or in the case of a high-risk pregnancy, labor. Upholding a light level of fitness may not be worth the extra and unexpected difficulties, culminating in obstacles to wellness. So while you enjoy the physical outlet, be smart about it!

Reminders regarding physical therapy, massage, and trainers:

1. Check with your insurance carrier before launching into physical therapy, massage, an exercise trainer and equipment, etc. Understand your options because hiring professionals is highly recommended; however, it may be too costly without partial insurance coverage.

2. Exercise at a regular time each day (ten to twenty minutes in the morning and the same in the afternoon; plug it into the Daily Schedule and do it!). Adding music helps make each session more enjoyable. Adding a friend is an ideal visit and provides a safeguard, someone present in the case of an unexpected issue.

3. If you are pregnant and bedridden, even the mildest exercise can cause contractions. Use extreme caution; it is recommended that you do not do squats, hold your breath, or exercise the muscles in the abdominal region.

Suggestions for simple exercises (doctor's approval needed first):

Deep breathing, yoga (not for pregnant patients),
Sitting or lying down, depending on your prescribed position, begin with ten deep inhalations and exhalations, holding each for five to eight seconds each. The breathing exercises help strengthen the chest muscles.

Isometrics
Isometric exercises can be done with any muscle group of the body. Depending on where your injury is, exclude the muscles in that sensitive area. In the case of pregnancy, don't use your abdominal muscles. Tighten and loosen each muscle group: face, neck, back, shoulders, arms, hands, thighs, calves, and feet. You may try to press your hands and feet against the headboard, footboard, or wall. Isometrics maintain circulation and muscle tone.

After the isometrics, loosen up each set of joints by rotating neck, shoulders, arms, hands, and feet.

Stretching
Remain in your prescribed bed rest position for all exercises:

Neck stretches—Tilt your head to the left as far as possible without strain, keeping shoulders level and relaxed, then tilt to the right side. Repeat ten times with each side.

Neck rotation—Keeping your shoulders level and relaxed, place your left hand on your left cheek, pushing gently with your hand while resisting slightly with your cheek. Turn your head as far to the right as you can, without strain. Reverse and use your right hand and your right cheek. Repeat ten times on each side.

Shoulder stretch—Raise your left shoulder toward your left ear as far as possible without tilting your head, then relax your shoulder completely and let it drop. Switch to the right side. Repeat two sets of ten with each side.

Shoulder roll—Roll both shoulders up and forward as high and as far forward as possible, then reverse. Do this six times each way.

Chest and Arms

Arm press—Lift your arms in front of you at right angles to your chest at nipple height. Bending your arms, press your palms together firmly. Push together and relax. Do two sets of ten.

Arm lift—Extend your arms fully out in front of you at about shoulder level, using either very light weights or canned goods of the same weight. With your arms still extended, lift your arms up slowly above your chest and head, and then back down toward the bed slowly. Repeat one to two sets of ten.

Biceps press—Holding the weights in your hands, and your arms extended fully in front of you at shoulder level, bend your arms at the elbows, bringing your hands to the shoulder, working the biceps. Repeat at least two sets of ten.

Wrist press—Extending your arms forward, palms up, hold weights in your hands, supporting the extended arms on pillows. Bend the arm at the wrist, bringing the hand toward the forearm as far as possible, holding the weights in the hand. Do one to two sets of ten, focusing on the forearms.

Handgrip—Use a handgrip, available at sporting good stores or online, or use a hard rubber ball, tennis ball, or racquetball. Squeeze as tightly as possible. You will build up your forearms.

Wrist rotation—Raise each arm and do wrist circles in each direction several times.

Leg lift—Turn onto your left side with your right leg stacked on top of your left leg, supporting your body with your right arm. Lift your right leg at a forty-five-degree angle with the foot flexed, pointing your toe slightly downward. Do two sets of ten. Repeat on the right side, lifting your left leg.

Ankle circles—On your side, lift your leg in the air and do circles with your ankle, flexing your foot as you come up and pointing your foot as you circle down. This is good for calf muscles. Repeat on the opposite side.

Hamstring and back combo stretch—Lying on your back, pull your left leg toward your chest. Keep the other leg as straight as possible, without straining. Do this on both sides. This will help to slowly loosen up the hamstrings and back muscles.

Whole leg stretch—On your back, bend your left knee, bringing your thigh to your abdomen, and then extend your left leg, flexing your foot. Keep the other leg as straight as possible. Hold your flex ten seconds or longer if you are comfortable and not straining. Repeat several times. Repeat with your right leg.

After you have completed your exercises, it is very important to do three things:

relax your whole body

breathe deeply, as if you were in a yoga class (slow and steady)

drink a large glass of water

Bed Rest, Exercise, and Sleep

Insomnia, a common issue for people with little or no physical activity, can be intensified by bed rest. Tension, anxiety, indigestion, or other discomforts can make it hard to fall asleep. If you are on medication around the clock, you may be forced to wake up several times during the night, which is not conducive to deep sleep. If you are in a different room than usual, or in a different bed, such as a rented hospital bed, sleeping soundly may be compromised.

Remedies to aid in relaxation before bedtime

warm milk

a light snack

a warm shower (if allowed)

a heating pad or hot water bottle in bed with you

a gentle massage

meditating

relaxing music

earplugs

Relaxation Techniques

Relaxing your mind and body is the best way to teach yourself how to fall asleep. Here are some techniques that experts have found particularly successful:

Slow down your breathing and imagine the air moving slowly in and out of your body while you breathe from your diaphragm.

Concentrate on relaxing your body one part at a time. Start with your toes, your feet, and your ankles, and work your way up. Go slowly.

Program yourself to turn off unpleasant thoughts as they emerge. To do that, think about enjoyable experiences that you've had. Reminisce about good times, fantasize, or play some mental games.

Avoid the following:

Stimulants after sunset (coffee, tea, sodas, chocolate, smoking);

Unnecessary medications that interfere with sleep (discuss this with your doctor if you suspect your medication is causing sleeplessness);

Difficult phone conversations or discussions with family or friends;

Working yourself into a frenzy fearing that you won't fall asleep.

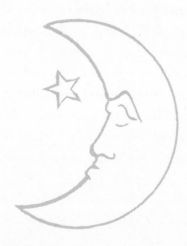

CHAPTER SIX

PICNICS IN BED

Nourishment and nurturance are two essential elements for all, but for people in a medically sensitive situation, their importance is magnified. For patients temporarily immobilized, nourishment becomes a basic form of nurturance. Therefore, consuming enough water and nutritious food is paramount for healing, and for overall health and happiness! Yet eating and drinking while you are immobilized is one of the biggest challenges. With a little creativity, the cooperation of helpers—family, friends, and caregivers—and a good sense of humor, the multitude of complications can be easily resolved.

Initially when bed rest is prescribed, your appetite may decrease, or you may feel like eating everything you can get your hands on due to generalized nervousness or fear of the unknown, or having low blood sugar due to unaccustomed inactivity. Creative solutions for eating, food preparation, storage, and accessibility have been thought out in this book, and help with getting started will enhance your level of comfort, motivation, and energy.

Liquids should be your first concern! Dehydration is your enemy as it can quickly cause illness and other medical complications. Also, dehydration can cause constipation, a problem closely associated with immobility. Prevention is resolved by drinking liquids (in the case of constipation, warm liquids are recommended, such as tea or hot water with lemon or juice). My first attempts at drinking liquids while lying flat were disastrous. Not only were the pillowcases and sheets instantly wet but it became unexpectedly irritating that someone else had to clean up after my constant spills. Discovering a lid-covered toddler cup and later, water bottles from my bike, resolved all frustrations! Eventually, I had color-coded water bottles for different fluids, a hand towel to dry spills, and a bib for extra security. Cycling water bottles became a mainstay for drinking all liquids: water, light juices, and vitamin- and electrolyte-enhanced water (I highly recommend coconut water, athletic performance formulas such as Cytomax, Endurox, ClifBar, or GU drink powders; one water bottle every three hours. They are all caffeine-free, with no sucrose or aspartame).

Try to drink at least eight glasses of water every day, even if getting up to use the toilet is forbidden or bothersome. Ask your medical team to help with this matter.

The art of "bed rest" food preparation, eating, cleaning, and storage is exciting! Certain foods work better than others. Eating my favorite baguette and pasta the first night was a disaster. The linguini swayed and sprayed marinara sauce everywhere, the crust of the baguette crumbled and showered onto the bed and inside my nightgown, even awakening me later in the night, and the little pieces of onion and carrots in my salad slipped off the fork causing stains on my blankets and pillows from the dressing! After a round of discussion with my husband, we agreed that in the future, the choice of pasta will be penne or shells or lasagna, salad will be put in a bowl that can be raised to my mouth, and softer bread will eliminate crumbs.

Uncomplicated foods need not be unimaginative foods. Wonderful combinations of cheese, meats, vegetables, spreads, and most anything else that you like, can be combined, spread or stuffed into breads, tortillas, or wraps. The possibilities are endless.

Eating nutritiously and efficiently is crucial to your healing process. You will play an important role in the foods you'll eat, but not your food prep. Your helpers will become experts in the art of bedside picnicking. If you hire a home-care service to do your shopping, meal preparation, and serving, make sure to communicate in writing how you prefer your meals. I favored eating small meals five to six times a day. I had a few personal demands, and I made them crystal clear to my husband and a few others: no salt or butter. I asked for a list of condiments for all meals, which my husband put into an attractive box to keep by my bed: honey, balsamic vinegar, seasoned rice vinegar, olive oil, mustard, pepper, dry chili peppers, cumin, cinnamon, powdered chocolate, and hand sanitizers. Being bedridden won't keep you from enjoying your favorite foods; it requires clear communication about what you want, how and when you want it, and mobilizing the right people to help with shopping, preparation, and serving.

Basic Principles and Requirements for Dining a la Bed Rest

Surroundings should be kept clean and organized.

An accessible, compact, and enclosed place for waste is necessary.

Constant and plentiful liquids.

Foods high in vitamins and minerals providing the most nutrition for the calories.

Foods rich in iron, calcium, magnesium, zinc, and the B-vitamin folic acid for building strength in healing and for pregnancy.

Fiber is more important than ever, especially for supporting digestion and preventing constipation.

Delegate your needs with clear communication, including how, when, and where for you and/or others (you may be delegating for others' meals i.e. small children, kitchen-disabled spouses, elderly dependents).

Sources of Recommended Nutrients:

Fiber: whole-grain cereals and breads, fresh fruits and vegetables, legumes, dried beans and peas, wheat-bran and oat-bran products.

Fluids: six to eight glasses of water or other non-caloric caffeine-free beverages daily in addition to milk, juice, smoothies, shakes.

Protein: fish, lean meat, poultry, eggs, beans, tofu, legumes, nuts, nut butters, protein powder.

Iron: lean red meats (beef, lamb, and pork), dark green leafy vegetables, canned sardines, fortified cereals, and grain products. To enhance absorption of iron from non-meat sources, combine them with other foods high in vitamin C, such as lemon juice, tomatoes, oranges, and other citrus fruits and juices.

Calcium: reduced-fat milk products such as milk, cheese, yogurt, frozen yogurt and ice milk, broccoli, kale, and other dark green leafy vegetables, canned sardines, and salmon (calcium comes from the edible bones).

Folic acid: oranges, orange juice, spinach, romaine lettuce, dark green leafy vegetables, beans, wheat germ, and nuts.

The Meal Setup

I preferred foods be delivered from the kitchen, especially at mealtime, and taken away when I was finished eating. I didn't like foods lingering on trays during the day, due to the smell, attracting flies, and my general desire for orderliness. This was not always possible, but I liked this concept the best. In my first bed rest experience, when I was one hundred percent confined and my husband left for work before I awoke and didn't return for at least ten hours, he developed a system for putting out my breakfast, lunch, and snacks in small coolers. Everything was labeled, and lined up where I could reach it. Each morning, the foods that I had requested the night before in a handwritten list for breakfast, lunch, and snacks were placed on my breakfast tray or in the coolers. This lineup also included a large hot water thermos so that there was always a choice between making hot tea, fresh brewed decaffeinated coffee, cocoa, or hot juice. My toddler cups and water bottles were always clean to begin each day, and initially filled for the first round of drinks. Extra water bottles, fresh ice in the cooler, and all of my snacks in containers or baggies were organized on the bedside table.

With the gamut of choices provided, I thrived on our innovative self-serve routine. After a while, it was hard to imagine normal life without the bedside cooler, the plastic baggie salad bar, the hand wipes, the small garbage container that was cleaned every day, and the dirty-dish container!

Supplies for Picnics in Bed

Lap tray

Bedside table even with mattress height

Ice chest with the daily staples such as a water jug; ice packs or bagged ice; condiments like butter, mayonnaise, mustard; salad dressing; peanut butter; perishable snacks such as carrot sticks, apples, oranges, lemons, string cheese

Water bottles, toddler cups with straws, personal thermos mugs

Utensils: fork, spoon, knife (three clean sets each day), cutting knife, small to medium-size cutting board, plate, bowl

Cloth napkins and dishtowels

Paper towels; keep roll at close reach

Condiment box

Dirty-dish container

Bib

Large hot water thermos or electric-coil water heater (must be connected to electrical outlet, which may require an extension cord, perhaps too difficult to maneuver)

Luxury items:

Small microwave on night table or bedside table already
plugged into outlet

Blender (optional—for liquid meals or smoothies)

Each day the utensils should be cleaned and replaced. All foods should be replenished. The thermos, bibs, water bottles, etc. should be emptied, rinsed, and dried for the next day of bed rest picnicking.

Meal Options

When faced with a situation like bed rest, it is easy to forget some of the most basic options for meals. In an attempt to help with simple yet delicious choices, I have organized suggestions by meal: breakfast, snacks, lunch, and dinner. Additionally, I have included lists of foods by nutritional category, e.g. proteins, iron-rich foods, etc. My hope is to encourage you to be creative and healthy for your eating pleasure and healing progress. Share your food and meal preparation ideas with your helpers and anyone else who will be cooking or preparing your meals. Otherwise you risk not being satisfied. You will see that once the job of shopping and preparing your foods is managed, you can easily enjoy a bed rest smorgasbord!

Breakfast

Instant hot cereal packages with fruit

Cereal with yogurt and fruit

Cottage cheese with fruit

Granola, yogurt, and soy milk with berries

Kasha (pilaf for breakfast, lunch, or dinner—sodium- and
cholesterol-free)

Eggs: soft- or hard-boiled, scrambled, poached with toast
and fruit

Tender asparagus makes a natural, edible utensil, delicious
alongside a cooked egg—dunk it into egg yolk, stir,
and eat.

Bagels and cream cheese; add lox, tomato, and onion, etc.

Waffles with maple syrup, honey, or fruit

French toast with maple syrup, honey, or fruit

Cinnamon toast and applesauce

Fruit salad and toast

Muffin or scone with yogurt and fruit (buy ahead baked goods
at your favorite bakery and freeze in plastic bags)

In an effort to maintain daily nutritional requirements, add yogurt, cheese, fruits, veggies, meat, or fish to your breakfast. Breakfast drinks are excellent sources of nutrition requirements; I recommend you start each day with something warm to drink for moving your digestive system: hot tea, coffee, cocoa, hot juice.

Nutritious Snacks

Deviled eggs

Celery with peanut butter and raisins

Sliced carrots, celery, radishes, and green onions—keep
fresh in cold water

Raw veggies: broccoli, cauliflower, red pepper, with a spread
or dip

Boiled baby red potatoes

Individual containers of yogurts, applesauce, dry soup

Dips: hummus, cream cheese and vegetable combinations,
peanut butter

String cheese, individually wrapped

Cheese and crackers

Sliced fruit: apple, pear, peach, orange, banana, melon, kiwi,
avocado (squeeze lemon over apple, avocado, banana,
and pear so they don't brown)

Nuts and raisins

Dried fruits (sulfide-free)

Cereal bars

Mixed cereals (i.e. granola, oat squares, raw oats, etc)

Rice cakes: plain or with cream cheese, peanut butter, apple
butter

Frozen fruit molds: cut up a variety of fruits, add lemonade
or

apple juice, and freeze in an ice cube tray or any other mold

Frozen yogurt: premix a container of yogurt and freeze
(vanilla, coffee caramel yogurts are especially delicious
this way!)

Frozen fruit: grapes, bananas, kiwi, mixed berries, pineapple

Popcorn

Crunchy pickles

Olives

Energy bars: made from whole grains and fruit. They are rich
in simple carbohydrates for quick energy, and complex
carbohydrates for sustained energy. This is an easy and
healthy way to refuel.

You may prefer to have four to six snacks during the day rather than a routine breakfast and lunch. This may be a better "system" if your kitchen help is limited. Simpler finger foods can be brought to your bed first thing in the morning (in abundance). Energy bars are an acceptable temporary solution for when resources are extremely limited. Awkward, sticky, soggy, or drippy foods do not work.

Lunch

Always balance your meal with a drink, fruit, protein, and
vegetable.

Soup in a thermos with baguette and cheese

Instant soup, preferably a preservative-free and low-sodium
brand (squeeze lemon into hot or cold soups to intensify
the flavor)

Bagel and cream cheese: add lox, salami, etc.

Fresh fruit salad: serve with yogurt or cottage cheese

Salad bar: mix together vegetables, fruit, cheese, raisins, nuts

Peanut butter and jelly sandwich

Tuna salad sandwich

Egg salad sandwich

Chicken or turkey salad sandwich

Ham and cheese sandwich

Grilled cheese sandwich

Pita with hummus or tuna, chicken, egg salad, etc.

Pizza

Quesadilla

Deli meats with pickles and cheese

Dry salami with cheese and crackers

Baked potato with sour cream or yogurt

Chili, cheese, and sour cream

Apple chunks with ham

Swiss cheese cubes and ham cubes on a skewer or toothpick

Beef and turkey jerky

Steamed (crisp) vegetables: broccoli, artichoke, beets, carrots, corn on the cob

Leftovers from dinner the night before

Keep a jar of salsa, chutney, jam, olive, pepper, basil pesto in your lunch cooler and enjoy more flavor on meat sandwiches, hot or cold, or with cheese and crackers.

Dinner

In the United States, dinner is traditionally the largest meal of the day and the more relaxed meal when family and friends eat together and socialize. While you are bedridden, simple dinners are ideal, and the chance to share meals with people is paramount. If you are confined to a wheelchair, you have the option of sitting at the dinner table. Whoever is doing the cooking should keep the focus on nutritious low-fat foods.

If your partner is cooking, try to keep the bed rest reality in perspective. Communicate gratitude. Your partner may not be used to cooking. Additionally, he or she may be tired from work, as well as concerned (stressed) about you, and pressured to create something fantastic to eat. The result may be that dinner, the more "important" meal of the day, is not as good as the other meals. Try to be patient. Encourage your helpers and emphasize simplicity. This way, no one can go wrong.

The following ideas for dinner preparation originate from my own experience with family and friends who successfully kept me well fed while bedridden for three months. Being in the wheelchair during my second round of confinement allowed me to prepare and cook a little bit for myself; however, I depended on these immeasurably helpful hints:

Make more than needed and freeze the extra!

Label everything, and, when possible, obtain defrosting and cooking instructions from the cook (use permanent marker and write directly on the wrapped food).

Using two or three master cooking efforts, diversify:

If someone makes a large batch of tomato sauce, store it for pasta, lasagna, chili, pizza, etc.

If a large amount of chicken is cooked, debone it, divide the meat, and save for making chicken pot pie, chicken enchiladas, chicken stew, chicken soup, chicken masala, chicken salad, etc.

Bake one large turkey or ham. Use the leftovers for sandwiches;

afterward, make a hearty soup from the remaining bone.

Double and triple casserole ingredients; cook and serve now, freeze the rest for many other meals.

Prepare large soups and stews; freeze and use for feeding visitors.

Steam vegetables slightly (crisp) and serve throughout the week.

Take the time to make a large fresh fruit salad, which can be served throughout the week.

Cookie dough can be frozen for more baking later.

A Basic Dinner
  I. Salad
 II. Main Course
III. Bread, Rice, or Potato
 IV. Dessert (optional)

Salad Ideas
mixed greens with onions, avocado, tomato, and carrots

romaine lettuce with parmesan cheese, croutons, and Caesar dressing

spinach, red onion, dried cranberries, goat cheese, roasted pinenuts, and rice vinegar/olive oil dressing

carrot salad with raisins, pineapples, mayonnaise, or yogurt dressing

butter lettuce with tangerines, green onions, and oil/vinegar dressing

Greek salad with feta cheese, olives, peppers, and lettuce

Main Course Ideas
pasta with sauce: tomato, pesto, alfredo, clams

sliced ham

sliced turkey

lasagna

stir-fried vegetables: add sauces to give it an ethnic flavoring (Indian curry, Chinese sesame oil, oyster sauce, Thai spices, etc.)

hearty soups and stews

baked potato stuffed with cheese, vegetables, meats

grilled fish

grilled or broiled sausages

meat: pork chops, lamb chops, steaks, chicken, veal

pizza: premade crusts make this very easy; try a variety of toppings such as pesto sauce, tomato sauce with goat cheese, green onions, sausage, eggplant, sundried tomatoes, etc.

chicken, turkey, or vegetable pot pie

meat loaf

burritos

Bread, Rice, or Potato Ideas

bread, breadsticks, pita, focaccia

rice: white, brown, wild, jasmine, basmati

potato: boiled, mashed, baked, french fries, etc.

risotto

pilaf, polenta, couscous

Dessert Ideas (optional)

fruit

tapioca or pudding cups

sorbet: bars or scooped in a dish

ice cream: bars or scooped in a dish

freshly baked goods, e.g. brownies, lemon squares, cookies, pie, etc.

Alternatives to Home Cooking

There will be many times when either no one is available or no one feels like cooking. There will also be times when you, your partner, your children, or a visiting friend prefers takeout. There is no better time than during this temporary period of confinement to take advantage of delicious restaurants and special preparation and delivery services.

For researching restaurants near you, go to Open Table, an online restaurant guide. There are also smartphone applications for restaurants by type of cuisine. You can also take on a mini-project by calling local restaurants and requesting that they send you their menus, and learning about their delivery options. It may help to explain your situation, and request that they make an exception for a local fan of their chef! Many different types of restaurants will help diversify and enhance your eating experience while bedridden. Each time I was bedridden, I craved the thought of sushi or Chinese food brought right to me!

Try These for Takeout
    Chinese
    Thai
    Laotian
    Vietnamese
    Cambodian
    Korean
    Italian
    Pizza
    Russian
    Mexican
    Mediterranean/Greek
    Ethiopian
    French
    Japanese/sushi
    Indian

California cuisine
Contemporary American
American delicatessen
Seafood

Liquids!

You cannot drink enough! Every chance you can get, drink a glass of water. Water transports nutrients to all parts of the body via the blood. It also serves as the medium for thousands of life-supporting chemical reactions constantly taking place in our bodies.

When I was on bed rest, I made a vow to drink between every "activity." Every time I went to the bathroom, got off the telephone, started a new project on the laptop, or ate something, I drank a glass of water. I encourage you to do the same.

cold water
mineral water (bubbly)
warm apple juice with cinnamon stick (extra source of
     vitamin C)
lemonade
tomato juice
prune juice
low-fat or nonfat milk
caffeine-free tea and coffee
fruit shake

Eliminate high-sugar drinks like sodas. Many are filled with caffeine, sugar, and aspartame. These substances will reduce your ability to feel well and focus on healing.

Nutrition Sources

Proteins

low-fat milk

low-fat or nonfat yogurt

frozen yogurt (freeze regular yogurt)

ice milk

buttermilk

cheese cubes

string cheese

grated cheese

parmesan

bags of crumbled blue, feta, farmer's cheese

hard-boiled or soft-boiled egg

tofu

textured vegetable protein (TVP)

nuts and seeds

wheat germ

freshwater fish

seafood

chicken

turkey

beef

lamb

pork

veal

legumes

peas

beans

lentils

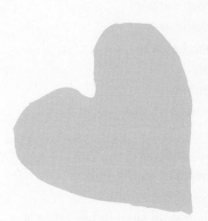

Vitamin C Foods

fruit and vegetable juices
orange
mango
papaya
apricots
cantaloupe
strawberries
blackberries
raspberries
blueberries
figs
tomatoes
cabbage
broccoli
green pepper
cauliflower
sweet potato
kale
kohlrabi
spinach

Calcium-Rich Foods

low-fat or nonfat milk
low-fat buttermilk
evaporated skim or low-fat milk
low-fat cottage cheese
cheddar or Swiss cheese
low-fat or nonfat yogurt
nonfat dry milk
orange juice

almonds

filberts

peanuts

dried fruit (sulfur-free)

canned salmon with bones

canned sardines with bones

sesame seeds

soy milk and soy protein

dark leafy greens

broccoli

figs

cooked beans

Iron-Rich Foods

dried fruit (sulfur-free is best)

beef

duck

liver

oysters (don't eat raw)

sardines

potatoes in their skin

spinach

seaweed

legumes (green peas, chickpeas, kidney and lima beans,
    lentils)

soybeans and soy products

blackstrap molasses

carob flour and carob powder

Vegetables
    asparagus
    green beans
    sugar snap peas
    jicama
    red, yellow, green bell peppers
    cucumbers
    brussels sprouts
    mushrooms
    okra
    zucchini
    broccoli
    carrots
    corn
    beets
    artichokes
    celery
    arugula
    onion

Supplements
    fish oil
    vitamin B12

Why Choose Organic?

I recommend choosing organic for all of your food and drink choices, with better taste being an easy and obvious explanation, yet here's exactly why:

Shop Organic—Save Energy

American farms have changed drastically in the last three generations, from the family-based small businesses dependent on human energy to large-scale factory farms highly dependent on fossil fuels. Modern farming uses more petroleum than any other single industry, consuming twelve percent of the country's total energy supply. More energy is now used to produce synthetic fertilizers than to till, cultivate, and harvest all the crops in the United States. Organic farming is still mainly based on labor-intensive practices such as weeding by hand and using green manures and crop covers rather than synthetic. Organic produce also tends to travel a shorter distance from the farm to your plate.

Eat Organic—Keep Chemicals Off Your Plate

Many pesticides approved for use by the EPA were registered before extensive research linking these chemicals to cancer and other diseases had been established. Now the EPA considers that sixty percent of all herbicides, ninety percent of all fungicides, and thirty percent of all insecticides are carcinogenic. A 1987 National Academy of Sciences report estimated that pesticides might cause an extra 1.4 million cancer cases among Americans over their lifetimes. The bottom line is that pesticides are poisons designed to kill living organisms, and they are also harmful to humans. In addition to cancer, pesticides are implicated in birth defects, nerve damage, and genetic mutations.

Choose Organic—Protect Farm Workers' Health

A National Cancer Institute study found that farmers exposed to herbicides had a six time greater risk of contracting cancer than those not exposed. In California, reported pesticide poisonings among farm workers has risen an average of fourteen percent a year since 1973, and doubled between 1975 and 1985. Field workers suffer the highest rates of occupational illness in the state. Farm worker health is also a serious problem in developing nations, where pesticide use can be poorly regulated. An estimated amount of one million people are poisoned annually by pesticides.

Shop Locally—Help Small Farmers

Although more and more large-scale farms are making the conversion to organic practices, most organic farms are small independently owned and operated family farms of less than one hundred acres. It's estimated that the United States has lost more than 650,000 family farms in the past two decades.

Choose Organic—Support a True Economy

Although organic foods might seem more expensive than conventional foods, conventional food prices do not reflect hidden costs borne by taxpayers. Other hidden costs include pesticide regulation and testing, hazardous waste disposal and clean up, and environmental damage.

Choose Organic—Promote Biodiversity

Mono-cropping is the practice of planting large plots of land with the same crop year after year. While this approach tripled farm production between 1950 and 1970, the lack of natural diversity of plant life has left the soil lacking in natural minerals and nutrients. To replace these nutrients, chemical fertilizers are used, often in increasing amounts.

Eating, shopping, and supporting organic is "the better way" for you, the environment, and the overall process of healing!

In summary, endless studies have documented the health benefits of organically grown food over non-organically grown food, not just because of the absence of chemical pesticides and herbicides, but for the levels of vitamins, minerals, and other micronutrients. There are much lower levels of nitrates, heavy metals, and other contaminants. Non-organic farmers most often fertilize their soil with only three components: nitrogen, phosphorus, and potassium, whereas organic farmers use a variety of fertilizers including compost, manure, and cover crops. Everything in the soil will be absorbed by the plant.

So when you buy organic produce you not only get chemical-free food, but you also get all the health benefits that rich, well-managed soil provides.

The foundation of organic agriculture is building and maintaining excellent soil. Soil management is a requirement under the National Organic Program, the Federal Organic Standards released by the USDA in 2002. Plants grown on healthy soil are much less susceptible to pests and so the need for pest eradication is reduced. Chemical-based agriculture, on the other hand, begins with soil that is already nutrient-depleted. And plants grown on depleted soil are weaker, more prone to disease and pests, and they need more chemicals!

Organic farming doesn't just protect the soil. It also protects other resources as well, such as water. Rich organic topsoil has a huge water-holding capacity so less water is needed for irrigation. In addition, by not using harmful chemicals on the farm, waterways, rivers, and streams are kept cleaner.

Systems that integrate the environment, the economy, and social concerns in a way that can be maintained in a healthy state indefinitely can be defined as sustainable. Therefore, a sustainable agriculture must be economically viable, socially responsible, and ecologically sound. In terms of food production, a sustainable agriculture cannot use up resources (soil, water, labor, community support, etc.) faster than it can (re)produce them. On the other hand, any type of agriculture that uses up or degrades its natural resource base, or pollutes the natural environment, will, over time, lose its ability to produce food and fiber.

At the same time, agriculture that isn't profitable will drive farmers out of business. What this means is that agriculture that fails to meet the needs of both the environment and society cannot be sustained.

Eat Organic—The Flavor Is Simply Better!

There's a good reason many chefs use organic foods in their recipes. The foods simply taste better!

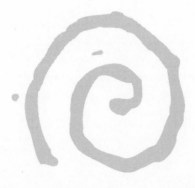

CHAPTER SEVEN

TECHNOLOGY AND BEING CONNECTED: A GUIDE TO SOCIAL MEDIA NETWORKS

No One Need Be Isolated!

When we are prescribed bed rest, it can feel scary and isolating. Humans are social creatures, and with this news, we may worry that being immobilized sets the stage for a period of loneliness and boredom. Thanks to the Internet, there are plenty of ways to connect, entertain, energize, and educate—whether it be yourself, a loved one, or a patient—ensuring that what initially seems restrictive is actually an opportunity for a productive, enriching experience.

You may have noticed various technology suggestions offered throughout this book. This particular section contains the same information but in one place, and in a little more detail. It is intended to be your "portable guide" to wireless Internet, laptop computers, e-readers, cellular phones and pertinent applications. While this technology has become an everyday part of many people's life experience, it is especially helpful when confronted with any type of physical immobilization or bed rest.

Note: This section is meant to be a basic guide, not an exhaustive manual, a jumpstart for immediate assistance and further exploration.

Getting Connected

While all of us used to be tied to a phone line, a bulky desktop, and a modem in order to access the Internet, now there are multiple ways to connect and use the Internet right from your bed, desk, and most other places! Listed below are portable methods for getting connected, and the pros and cons of each so that you can determine which works optimally for your unique situation.

Voice transcription software: As typing can be physically difficult for some who are bedridden, exploring the option of voice transcription software is recommended. This allows you to speak into a microphone inside your laptop, phone, or other device, which prompts your words to be typed out for you. This technology exists in new smartphones. There are various applications such as "Dragon" which can be obtained for free or a small cost online.

Windows versus Macintosh: There are two main operating systems for computers: Mac (by Apple) and Windows (by Microsoft). People tend to prefer one over the other for various reasons, and both have their advantages and disadvantages. I recommend you explore reviews and consumer comparisons (online or in related magazines) to get more details about which one fits you or the user. Windows-based computers tend to require more software to protect them from viruses. Mac computers are less likely to fall under attack or to crash (meaning to freeze or turn off randomly).

Laptops: Luckily they have gone from a luxury item to an everyday appliance. Most have the same processing power as a desktop. New laptops tend to range from five hundred to two thousand dollars, so do your research! If possible, borrow and test one to see if you like how it performs, before you purchase your own. For example, if you want to watch videos on your laptop, play the newest games, or download large files, this will require a laptop with a faster processing speed than if you only use it for email and social media like Facebook or Twitter. CNet.com is one of the places I use to compare and contrast technology.

Netbooks: Designed to be mini-laptops, they are made to be ultra-portable:

lightweight, powerful, and easy to use. They tend to lack "extra" features such as a CD or DVD player or expanded memory. (That's not a big deal, as you can plug-in extras as needed.) Netbooks tend to run in the two-hundred-and-fifty to five hundred dollar range, but remember they may be slower and have a smaller keyboard, which is complete but handles differently. They are ideal for the person who primarily wants to access email, social media, blogs, and other low-processing data.

Tablets: They function very similarly to netbooks. The usual tablet computer form is called a *slate*—a touch screen with a virtual keyboard on the screen itself. Because it is less bulky and easy to use with one hand, a tablet can be just right for people confined to a bed. However, because of the constant touching of the screen, there is a likelihood it could get damaged, or that overuse may cause undesirable neck, shoulder, or wrist tension. Tablets are often easier for watching videos, reading books online, or drawing, as you will use a finger or a stylus to directly navigate the pointer (rather than indirectly via a mouse or touchpad). If you don't intend to do a lot of typing, a tablet is a helpful tool.

Smartphones: Thse tiny tools have become extremely popular in the last few years as they are like compact computers. Smartphones have Internet access both by wi-fi and via the cellular phone networks, allowing you to telephone *and* surf the web anywhere. Some smartphones have built-in keyboards; others have virtual keyboards. I recommend that you review the latest smartphone options to determine what works best for your situation, with consideration for your location and access to cell coverage and wi-fi. Smartphones range in price, and can be purchased with or without a provider contract. Watching videos, answering emails, and checking social media can be achieved with a smartphone. Websites may not be easy to navigate on a smartphone.

Netiquette: How to Get Along

Interacting via the Internet is similar to real life communications; we are more productive when positive, polite, succinct, and mindful. Without body language or eye contact, online communication can easily be misinterpreted; therefore, a few basic principles can ensure your time online is pleasant and productive:

Even though the Internet is anonymous, manners go a long way (many people toss them to the wayside).

Use common sense, such as avoiding inflammatory language, and if someone seems rude, "walk away." You don't have to engage with anyone or any content you don't want to.

When appropriate, begin contact with a simple greeting, even if you do not include individual names, for example: Hello! Greetings! Hi there! This sets a friendly tone without being overly personal. Sign off or end with a closing, such as: Thank you, Cheers, Best to you, Take care, Will be in contact soon.

Forums

Before I start to talk on a forum, I like to lurk beforehand, reading what other people have posted to get a feel for the way people interact. Are they warm and friendly? Are there topics they avoid (like politics and religion)? Do they enjoy respectful debate?

By understanding the feel of the site or forum, it becomes easier and more effective to immerse yourself in the culture.

One great way to get started is to ask a few questions, or answer other people's questions. Sharing what you know or have experienced demonstrates that you're "there" to give as well as take, and everyone likes that! While these venues aren't formal, it's a good idea to take advantage of available typing assistance: use a spellcheck, read and edit what you've written before clicking "post." Be aware too that typing in all capital letters translates online to shouting.

Don't forget to spend time offline! It can be easy to lose hours staring into a computer monitor catching up on Facebook or involving yourself with forums. There is software that helps limit overuse of personal time on the computer, and it can be installed!

A QUICK GUIDE TO NETSPEAK

AFK away from keyboard

ASAP as soon as possible

BRB be right back

BTW by the way

FYI for your information

IDK I don't know

IMHO/IMNSHO in my humble opinion/in my not-
so-humble opinion

LOL laugh out loud

OMG oh my god!

TTYL talk to you later

XOXO kisses and hugs

A Note on Spam and Viruses

The Internet is not always a nice, friendly place. Be aware that clicking on links or downloading attachments from people you don't know can lead to your computer being attacked by a virus and/or used to send unsolicited emails called spam to everyone in your address book. Most devices have built-in spam filters to avoid those messages getting through, but proceed with caution if you are sent emails or chat messages from strangers.

Social Media and Micro-blogging

Social media, also called micro-blogging due to the relative briefness of the posts, has become the village square for the new millennium. With multiple ways to communicate with friends, reach out to people from the past, and meet new people, social media can be an appealing way to find out what's going on. Different styles of interaction appeal to different people—pick one that works for you.

Twitter, with its text limit of 140 characters, is known for being the place to keep up with celebrities, politics, companies you like, and to see what friends and colleagues have been doing. You can post your own updates, follow updates from other users, and send public or private messages. Twitter is also a way to text people internationally. Now that many people have smartphones, you can set up messages called "tweets" to go directly to your phone to help you keep in touch. Mashable.com/guidebook/twitter provides an in-depth idea of how to best use social media.

Facebook is the place to keep in touch with family, friends, and people with similar interests all around the world. This site allows you to post photographs and videos, follow interesting links, and play online games. You can even instant message people through Facebook! Unlike other social media sites, Facebook provides the option for privacy, including sharing individual photo albums, posts, and personal exchange of information. Cnet.com is a great place to start to learn more about this network.

Tumblr is a blogging website focused mainly on one or two paragraphs of comments and images of various kinds. There are tumblrs devoted to a variety of specific interests such as fashion, recipes, animals, and politics. When you start a tumblr, you can re-blog posts you find interesting and share them with your followers. The main page on Tumblr is called a dashboard, and on your dashboard, you'll see all the updates from the various tumblrs you follow, allowing you to quickly browse multiple posts from multiple people. It is an efficient and fun way to discover new things.

Other popular sites are Google +, Pinterest.com and Path. Explore these sites and further connect with friends and family.

Community

While micro-blogging is great for quick exchange and exposure to information and ideas, you may want to go into more depth. Blogs and forums offer a close-knit community where you can obtain support and advice, and, of course, offer your own experience to help others.

Specialty forums, which are based around specific topics, are great ways to connect with people with similar interests. Begin by searching forums of your own interest, and you will see that most allow you to read posts without needing to create a username or a password. Others may require you to sign in, and create a password. Hospitals have their own forums for patients and families of patients to interact with each other; ask your local facility about their forums. Additionally, you will find specific forums about specific situations, such as pregnant mothers who have been prescribed bed rest, or people managing life in a wheelchair, or others having to be reclined over an extended period of time. Check out "Care2," a global forum for activists of many specific subject matters. If you search for a forum on a special interest, chances are there is a forum for it!

While keeping a diary is a great idea, especially while immobilized, there are options of how to go about doing this, and one is to keep a journal or diary online. Various blog platforms support privacy, and if you want to share your entries with only select people, you can invite others to subscribe to your blog. A blog can also be public. The easiest free blogging platform is WordPress. It allows customized styling. All online journals offer the opportunity for freedom and space to be creative as well as entirely honest about the triumphs and tribulations of your experiences. Another advantage of personal blogs is the ability to review and reflect, to look back on where you were months and even years earlier and where you are today, all by maintaining an easy-to-use archive of your words.

LiveJournal is one of the largest places for bloggers to gather and talk. Anyone can create a free personal blog and write about whatever strikes their fancy. A highlight feature of LiveJournal is the ability to join communities and have posts from those communities show up on your friends' pages. This is one way to obtain specialty advice from current or past posts that may be relevant.

Online Films and Videos

Being on bed rest means no going to the movies, and depending on where you are resting, you might not have access to cable television. But there are lots of ways to take a break with some film or video entertainment right from your bed, sofa, or desk, using the Internet:

Free TV—Many television channels have an online presence allowing you to view their more popular shows through their website; some also offer access to news broadcasts. In addition, there are sites like Hulu.com where many shows are archived and available to view on demand. This allows you to pause a show so you can do other things and then resume when it's convenient for you.

Netflix and Amazon Prime are the top subscription services for which you pay monthly in exchange for access to all types of films. Additionally, you can have DVDs mailed to your house, or you can watch a slightly smaller selection of media immediately on your device though Netflix's player. They both offer a first month discount so you can explore their service, trying it before you buy it.

YouTube is an online site for people to upload, share, and view videos, from fan music videos and short animations to documentaries and how-to's. While often dismissed as a place to watch silly videos, there is a large selection of available informational material as well. For example, if you want to learn some new makeup skills, or how to knit, or if the patient desires pesto and you've never made this before, you can search for videos on YouTube that will demonstrate these techniques.

Online Books

If you are a voracious reader, and the library or shopping at a bookstore is not currently an option, never fear. There are superb resources online to give you hours of reading material, right at your fingertips:

E-readers, or electronic reading devices, are lightweight and slender and provide hundreds of books at your fingertips. The two most common brands are the Kindle, which only works with Amazon.com downloads, and the Nook, which is available through Barnes & Noble. The Kindle has a variety of editions (from simple to more options and power), a keyboard and is wireless, while the Nook utilizes a touch screen. The Nook has the option of the "LendMe" feature, which lets you "lend" a book to a friend for up to a week. You may find an e-reader easier to manage than physical books while bedridden.

Project Gutenberg is the oldest digital library, and archives cultural works that are public domain and now available for free online. This is how to catch up on the classics, with the works of Charles Dickens, Jane Austen, H. G. Wells, and many more.

Online magazines: If you love reading but books are less your style, check out online magazines. The new e-readers offer full access to hundreds of magazines. Magatopia is an online site that has thousands of magazines available, often for free. One advantage to online magazines is that they can link to earlier issues, allowing you to follow a topic and read opinions by different journalists.

Good Reads/Library Thing/Paperback Swap: There are ways to use the Internet to access new and used physical books. Good Reads and Library Thing are online services to catalogue books, and you can sign up to be an early reviewer of new releases. Paperback Swap is an online marketplace where you can trade your old books to other people who are also trading books. A vast variety of accessible literature is at your fingertips.

Staying Connected, Meeting and Making Friends

Skype is a popular voice over Internet Protocol (VoIP) service. Google Chat also has a video option, as do various Apple products via FaceTime. These services allow you to call and chat with another person for free. Skype enables you to call a landline or mobile phone for a cheaper rate than most phone services. Being able to have video chats with friends and family helps everyone feel more connected.

MMOs (massively multiplayer online games) are games you can play online where you can interact with other people from all over the globe. Many people find MMOs to be great for meeting people and keeping their minds active when on bed rest. Online games where you create an avatar and use it to explore your environment are stimulating ways to spend time, but be cautious, it can be all too easy to get lost in the game and forget about the outside world! Use a timer if you might be inclined to over-use.

Free online games: If large game universes don't interest you, there are also ways to play Scrabble, chess, backgammon, and other board games online. Facebook offers online games, ranging from strategy games to simple "timewasters." There are also games such as Kingdom of Loathing, which is a primarily text-based strategy game, or Echo Bazaar, a low-graphics game. Both of these limit the number of turns you can take per day, preventing overuse. (A quick warning: Games are made to be addictive, avoid overuse.)

Personal Productivity as an Opportunity for Income

For those who are immobilized or bedridden, personal income may be reduced during this time of recovery. A desire to continue to earn money while unable to go to work can turn new experiences/personal projects into a moneymaking venture. There are multiple ways to use your time productively, and when personal productivity becomes an opportunity for income, it can take some of the sting out of needing to take time off work.

Consumer reviews: Various companies seek consumer reviews, in exchange for honest, unbiased review of products. You can be one of the reviewers! Additionally, creating a blog where you review products under a uniting banner such as "Nursing Products for New Mothers" or "The Green Guide to Home Health and Rehabilitation" can pass the time while also becoming a business venture.

Marketing research: Companies pay for responses to product surveys. The surveys can take from five to fifty minutes, and can be done through various websites or via email, right on your computer.

YouTube, Etsy, etc.: Your personal projects, crafts, arts, and hand-hewn products can be exhibited and sold on websites, such as Etsy. When you research the options, you will find that for very little investment, you can have an online presence, a storefront, and sales! You can even use YouTube to learn a new skill, and then craft things to sell online, allowing you to stay busy, entertained and make a tidy sum on the side.

Conclusion

Bed rest can be a fantastic opportunity for personal growth and a whole new life-style. While it is an invitation to relax and take some time for yourself away from the bustle of everyday life, it is also a time to learn new skills, and to engage your brain in a new way. Using the Internet productively and mindfully reduces the feeling of isolation because it offers so many interesting opportunities to connect with family, friends, and associates, meet new people, be creative, and explore ideas! It is a superb tool not only for communication, but for improving yourself and enriching life while enduring a medical challenge.

Resource List

The easiest way to find these websites is to type in the title of the article or page listed here in the search box at google.com.

Netiquette and text speak

A Guide to Internet Lingo and Emoticons—PC World
pcworld.com/article/88686/lol_a_guide_to_internet_lingo_
and_emoticons.html

Twitter Dictionary Guide—Webopedia
webopedia.com/quick_ref/Twitter_Dictionary_Guide.asp

Twitter Slang—No Slang
noslang.com/twitterslang.php

List of Chat Acronyms & Text Message Shorthand—Netlingo
netlingo.com/acronyms.php

Social media and micro-blogging

Facebook, Twitter, and Tumblr:
Follow micro-blogs by using the tag bed-rest or immobility

Twitter accounts for pregnancy-related bed rest:

@Makingthemostofbedrest
@bedrestwellness
@KeepEmCookin
@TheChattyMomma
@mamasonbedrest

Community—resources and advice about being on bedrest
> bedrestwellness.com
> keepemcookin.com
> pregnancy.about.com
> embracebedrestblog.com/category/sanity-savers/

Get some ideas on crafts you can explore at the tumblr blog Craftspiration.
> craftspiration.tumblr.com/

Check out some travel photography on the tumblr blog Travel This World.
> travelthisworld.tumblr.com/

Have a good laugh at the blog Hyperbole and a Half.
> hyperboleandahalf.blogspot.com (humor blog)

Online videos and books
> Check out how-to videos at Howcast.com.
> YouTube.com also has many tutorials on a variety of subjects; learn a new language, get some makeup skills, or try a new craft!
> Hulu.com offers a lot of television shows online for free.

> PaperbackSwap.com or GoodReads.com are excellent websites for people who prefer physical books to trade and review them.

Staying connected through games
> mmohuts.com/
> techcult.com/the-150-best-online-flash-games/

Recycle, donate, or trade things you're no longer using, from magazines to equipment.
> freecycle.org/

Personal productivity as a source of income
> etsy.com/ (buy and sell handmade, vintage, and supplies)
> epinions.com/ (write product reviews)
> amazon.com (write product reviews)
> helium.com/write_menu (write reviews, get paid)
> contributor.yahoo.com/signup/ (write reviews, get paid)
> fiverr.com/ (hire people to do things for five dollars)

The power of exercise and bed rest
> thepowerofexercise.com
> nextstepfitness.com/fitness-dvds/bedrest-fitness-dvd.html
> ehow.com/how_2285905_exercise-bed-rest.html

CHAPTER EIGHT

PERSONAL PROJECTS

Keeping busy is good therapy for all people, but especially good for those who are immobilized. For most people who are bedridden or confined to a wheelchair or couch, mixing activities helps energize each day. There is time to adventure into quiet projects, for instance, to rediscover an old hobby or explore a new one. My suggestions carry the intention of exciting your curiosity, creativity, and productivity. Some of these ideas may catch you by surprise—something you wouldn't think to explore but this reminder ignites an interest or another idea. Please do not deny yourself any activity if it sounds gender specific. Being absorbed and creative is wonderful; being open is part of the fun, and key to faster healing. Have a great time being stimulated while staying quiet!

Your bed and the room in which you spend most of your time should be accessible to family and friends, but also a place where being private, quiet, and still is given the utmost priority. It should not be a place that is too loud or invites so much activity that you become hyper or anxious. You and your community must understand and respect the limitations of your medical state, before you invite them to jump in and have a great time.

Along these same lines, the room should be childproof so that togetherness is encouraged; everyone can maximize visits and not worry about potential disasters.

Bed Games

Ideas for playing games independently or with others of any age are below. Many games can now be enjoyed via the computer and cell phone. Games that are played on the bed should be lightweight, should not require physical effort, or contain spillable liquids. Research "board games" online for more of a selection. For books on this subject, go to amazon.com, and search on books/family games. There is an endless supply of fun awaiting you!

Board games

Scrabble

Monopoly

Trivia

Candy Land

Clue

Yahtzee

Checkers

Backgammon

Chess

Chinese checkers

Mancala

Jigsaw puzzles

Crossword puzzles

Cards

Other Kinds of Play!

Coloring books

Modeling clay

Model building

Reading joke books (laughter is one of the best medicines available!)

Reading riddle books

Viewing videos or special television shows

Group reading (plays, storytelling, short stories, novels, newspaper)

Hugs and tickling (very small children love the "Tickle Monster")

Strings games such as Cat's Cradle

Finger songs, ("Itsy-Bitsy Spider," "London Bridge")

Finger puppets, puppet dolls, puppet shows

Hand shadows

Reading and Studying

There are a variety of formats to read from beyond just paperbacks or hardcovers—you can enjoy e-readers such as Kindles and iPads.

Books by the same author

Books by genre, e.g. romance, mystery, poetry, fiction, science fiction; and nonfiction: biography, psychology, self-help, health, business, childcare, history, pop culture, career development

Your child's schoolbooks

Books on your bookshelf, purchased and never touched

Newspapers and magazines (daily, weekly, monthly/online or home delivery)

Domestic and international newspapers

Health and wellness

Science journals

Nature

Automobile

Craft

Architecture and design

Sports: running, triathlon, yoga, adventure, sailing, etc.

Technology

Travel

Travel, maps, atlas

Cookbooks

Cartoons, jokes, riddles

Baby names

Local history

Family tree

Old letters

Medical books on your physical condition or other areas of interest

Coursework or correspondence courses: work toward a new degree

Recorded books: Recorded Books, Inc. provides unabridged single-voice performances on book-packaged cds featuring the very best books in and out-of-print, available for both rental and purchase, by mail or download. (For more information and a free catalog, call 800-638-1304 or www.recordedbooks.com or www.audible.com.)

Writing

Personal Journal

Writing is a terrific way to express thoughts and feelings, especially now. My bed rest journals contain random thoughts, reminders, to-do lists, creative writing pages, phone numbers, and scribbles from each experience. Even though I had my laptop nearby, journal writing by hand was different, and helped me through some hard times, some very intense feelings, and many hours of being alone. When I had emotional dips, I often turned to my bed rest journal. Each time, the upset quickly dissipated. After medical exams, when there was positive news, I wrote in my journal for the overflow of happiness. Processing feelings through writing helped me get through the varied terrain of bed rest. Additionally, recording medical updates in a notebook is important, and may provide a significant reference at different doctors' offices, thus handwriting in your own medical journal is wise. I encourage you to keep a journal. It will be a treasure to read months and years later.

Postcards, Letters, Notes

Handwriting a postcard, letter, or note to your partner, children, new baby, other family members, friends, and work associates is a great way to communicate. Hand-written messages are few and far between these days, and have a special effect. Additionally, words of appreciation and expressions of love will make you and others feel good.

Creative Writing on the Laptop, iPad, Paper notepad

A very satisfying activity is authoring your own short stories, screenplays, comics, poems, songs, novels, letters-to-the-editor, political commentary, letters to a pen pal. Also, contributing to a charitable organization by addressing envelopes is wonderful as well as learning the art of calligraphy.

JOURNAL SAMPLES

February 17, 2012

Two weeks of bed rest has passed and I am surviving. I could never have imagined myself being able to endure this for more than a day but it's not that terrible. The key for me is to stay busy and I'm somehow able to find things to occupy my time. I find I enjoy organizing with a lot of details! Lots of things to do, things that the house needs and ideas for gifts for people with birthdays. Oh god, my life is mundane. At least the laptop is figured out so I can use email which eats up a lot of time. The work thing makes me very tired. I'm not sure how long I can maintain my focus.

I love my shower even if it's only twice a week. The hot water feels so good on my body, but five minutes isn't long enough, but beggars can't be choosey. Bed rest is not going to kill me. It's going to be tough, that's a lot of days ahead of me, but there's no choice. I like when people visit, but I also like just being alone. The visitor thing – it sends me 'up' and then when I say goodbye, I feel my isolation intensely. Maybe it's easier if no one comes? What helps is to get quickly absorbed in a video, phone call, knitting, or reading. I'm trying hard to keep my chin up. I've got to be strong.

February 28, 2012

It was a sunny today. The blossoms are in full bloom right outside my window. I wish I could dance around outside. No way this Spring. I'm a little down today. I literally have to force myself to accept being bedridden and focus on the physical therapy exercises, reading good books, preparing my snacks from the "snack bar" on my bed, and remembering that I have lots of support. I wish I didn't get so hungry—I don't want to blow up while being so inactive. O.K., no more fattening foods in my cooler and no treats, even though everyone who comes by gives affection via good food! I need new eating habits, I guess this is the time to practice control?

Crafts

Needlework

This kind of craftwork is great for keeping hands active, and minds and eyes focused on something colorful and rewarding. There's nothing like a finished product, either enjoying it yourself or giving it as a gift (a crocheted afghan; hand-knit hat, sweater, or vest; beaded bracelets and necklaces; macramé belts or wall hangings, etc). Depending on the project, others can join you. Pace yourself so as to avoid hand, arm, or wrist strain.

Knitting: Whether knitting colorful squares for a baby blanket, coordinated vests for the entire family, a complicated Norwegian ski sweater, socks, hats, or new Christmas stockings, this craft is very rewarding.

Sewing: Choose something that can lie out in front of you, that isn't too complicated, and allows for hand sewing (small portable sewing machines may work depending on your position). Sewing small items is recommended such as dolls, dolls' clothing, skirts, shorts, shirts, ties, quilts, scarves, etc.

Needlepoint: You can make pillows, a picture for the baby's room, bookmarks, eyeglass cases, or a sign that says, "sleeping," to hang over the doorknob of your own bedroom. This is a very pleasant activity.

Stitchery: Kits are available at most craft centers. A hoop to brace the material is highly recommended to reduce strain on arms and hands.

Embroidery: A fine needle and colorful thread allow you to transform napkins, tablecloths, shirts, jeans.

Crocheting: With a skein of yarn and one small hook, you'll be amazed how quickly you can create something useful. Crocheted afghans, hats, headbands, and vests are fashionable right now. This is probably the easiest needlework and least strain on your arms and hands.

Rug hooking: Latch-hook rugs are easy and lightweight. You can hook by hand or with a special hook. This is something you can do with the help of others.

Handcrafts

Beadwork: The possibilities are endless with beads. To get started, you can use dental floss and a sewing needle. Elastic string is ideal for making necklaces, bracelets, anklets, earrings, hairpieces, etc. With other materials, such as jeweler's wire and proper tools, you can design and create earrings, bracelets, and necklaces with the finest of gems, medals, pearls, and stones. Buttons, pieces of worn glass, letter cubes, shells, raw pasta, and large and small beads can be beaded alone or with others. Important advice: Keep all beads in containers so that you do not end up sharing your bed with them.

Model making: From cars to horses, the possibilities are endless. Make sure your room is well ventilated if you are using glue or epoxy.

Candle making: Small or large candles can be easily created with the right procedure. Explore adorning your creations with strips of colorful wax, cutout shapes, and textured designs. Natural or colored beeswax candles are easy and offer a divine fragrance. Candles make nice gifts or additional decoration for your room.

Macramé: This activity is a creative outlet and superb for arm and hand exercise. You can make belts, dog or cat collars, planters, jewelry, wall hangings, and more.

Woodworking: Woodworking with small pieces of wood is advisable only if you have experience with tools and carving wood. A friend, pregnant with her first child who landed in the hospital for weeks with complications, made a baby stepstool by sanding precut pieces and painting and varnishing it (all while lying in bed). A male friend, who was immobilized due to vascular inflammation in his legs, made beautiful woodcuts from his wheelchair. The carving, inking, and printing were all done from a worktable set up for other craft projects. Suggestions for wood carving: Use sharp utensils with great care and only if you have a lot of previous experience; use a plastic bag under and over your body to prevent wood chips from getting inside your clothing or bed. If you are pregnant, consult with your doctor before using glue, varnish, or other materials that might have toxic fumes.

Good Resources for Crafts

    craftsolutions.com

    craftideas.info

    allfreecrafts.com

    marthastewart.com

    craftgossip.com

    thriftyfun.com

    favecrafts.com

Art

When else would you ever have this much privacy or time to express yourself artistically? Have you ever experimented with art, enjoyed it, felt very satisfied, and then never followed through to explore your talent? Have you ever had the urge to drop everything for a while and tap into your creative gifts? Now is your chance.

Drawing: What could be simpler? You will need plain paper or a sketchpad, pencils, and an eraser. Add to your possibilities with colored pencils, crayons, watercolors, charcoal, paints, and small canvases. Good sources for materials are local art stores, and for guidance, have someone pick up a drawing or painting guide at a nearby bookstore, art store, or library. You might try tracing family photos or magazine pictures. Fabric paint is an easy-to-use way to hand-decorate household items such as flower pots and glass vases or cups; put your personal touch on sweatshirts, T-shirts, shoes, baby bibs, dolls, lunchboxes, etc. Suggestion when using wet paints: Use a plastic garbage bag on the lap tray and either wear a plastic smock or put another garbage bag under your body to protect the bed.

Clay: Have someone deliver a good-size hunk of clay to your bedside. Always keep it in plastic to preserve the necessary moisture for kneading and sculpting. Whenever you feel like sculpting something, take it out and mold away. Jewelry and pottery can be made with Fimo dough and other ceramic clays. There are many good clay guidebooks. Some books include colorful clay samples. Get the specifics on how to maintain the clay so you don't get discouraged or waste time and money by using it incorrectly. Use a plastic garbage bag on the lap tray and either wear a plastic smock or put another garbage bag under your body to protect the bed. Be forewarned—many clays have a fairly strong odor. Hopefully this won't be a problem for you.

Photography: If self-processing photographs is something you've always wanted to do, invest this time in reading everything there is to know about the art and science of photography.

When you are mobile, you will be an expert, prepared and ready to set up a darkroom and apply your learned skills. While in bed, you can experiment with cameras and film, trying techniques and analyzing the effects by having the film processed elsewhere. There is so much that can be digitally processed using the computer and specialized software. You may also enjoy teaching yourself the art of color-tinting old black-and-white photos. To begin, ask someone to bring you black-and-white photocopies of a favorite photograph to practice and test your sense of color. When you are ready, collect actual photos and begin doing the real thing. You may find you have a side business in the making, perhaps while you are still bedridden.

Paper: Teach yourself origami, the art of paper folding. There are numerous resources online and excellent books, some of which include special paper for getting started. Making paper chains, paper airplanes, paper dolls, paper houses, paper snowflakes, paper cutouts of all kinds, is a fun way to spend time, especially with children. However, you don't have to have little ones around to enjoy paper art. Make your own note cards, postcards, and birthday cards. Suggestion: Use glue sticks rather than glue in a bottle. Do not use super glues unless your room is well ventilated.

Photo Albums

Scrapbooks and photo albums built by hand or online require few tools and promise to occupy one's attention for large blocks of time. They can be special keepsakes or gifts. Ideas for personal use or gifts: new baby album, family photo journal, special recipe album, and personal correspondence collection.

Best strategy:

> Collect all the photos, either gathering them online or physical copies.
>
> Organize by year, month, and day, theme, or person.
>
> Ask someone to buy scrapbooks, photo albums, or large binders of your choice; you should look online or in catalogs for what best fits your needs. Be specific regarding the size and capacity, format, and number of albums you'll need.
>
> Mount and label the photos. If there are "extras" and you do not want to discard them for sentimental reasons, cut out the essential parts of the photo (around someone's head and body or around a beautiful building or garden), and with ingenuity—collage style—whimsically decorate the album's page. This approach uses available space and offers fun viewing.

Music

It is never too late to learn how to play a musical instrument or to read notes. If you already play an instrument, and it's light enough to be held while you are immobilized, do it! If you normally play a large instrument, such as the drums or the cello, and there's no way to continue while on bed rest, try a ukulele or another small instrument. What about an electronic keyboard? It is narrow enough to fit next to you if you are on your side, or it can be placed on a lap tray. Keyboards are sold everywhere these days, including big box stores like Costco and Kmart. For beginners, basic music theory books and self-teaching books are available online and in local music stores. Words of caution: Playing an instrument takes a lot of energy, especially from a reclined position. Observe your breathing and heart rate, as you do not want to increase either to an undesirable point.

Listen to music on an iPod, cd player, or whatever device you have that fits by your bed or chair, and is easily self-operated. Consider obtaining good headphones while you are physically confined, that way the quality of the sound is superb, and your sounds do not interfere with anyone else. If you normally listen to one type of music, such as jazz, classical, or rap, consider expanding your auditory experience to country, hip-hop, or opera. Because you have the time and liberty, you may discover a whole new world of musical pleasure! Be aware of how certain genres increase your energy, and pay attention to your heart rate with specific types of music. It is ill advised to cause an elevation in either. On a personal note, I loved listening to bluegrass during my first pregnancy, but when I was bedridden, I had to dismiss the urge as it "energized" me and caused contractions.

On your laptop, phone, or iPod, continually create and update playlists for increased pleasure, inspiration, relaxation, and quality of life.

Attending to the Personal

Family History: Right now is an excellent opportunity to delve into your personal history. There are probably lost archives, genealogy charts, and an incomplete family tree waiting to be explored and updated. Networking for information and updating your history is a meaningful and rewarding venture. Call or write family members, use the Internet, and pursue and expand your ancestry.

Personal finances: Being confined to your home, apartment, or to a particular room (perhaps in the hospital or a hotel), invites the opportunity to venture into personal projects as well as other massive undertakings that you have desired or neglected to do. With long blocks of quietude, personal finance is waiting for your attention. Everything from finally learning online banking, to managing your budget and organizing receipts and tax paperwork can now be conquered. Now might be just the time to meet with your accountant, investment advisor, or a friend in the field, all of whom can visit with the purpose of enhancing your personal finances. Excellent resources available to further support this undertaking are the business section of newspapers, specific financial publications (*Wall Street Journal*, *The Economist*, books on money and finance, etc.), and banks' personnel.

Filing: Like personal finances, personal filing is typically neglected because it begs for focused attention, which requires blocks of time. Now is an ideal time to organize life's papers and passions: automobile ownership and maintenance, banking, credit cards, insurance policies, warrantee information for home and lifestyle accessories, keepsake newspaper articles, photos, correspondence, personal writing, legal matters, professional documents and résumé, travel journals and maps, home decorating ideas, house and property construction and renovation projects, etc.

Personal and private (time): There is barely enough time in life to do what we need to do, therefore, having idle time can be strange for most people. Why not take these moments as an opportunity? Just do the personal things you never before had time for, such as:

   Trim your own hair (prior experience advised)
   Have a stylist visit for a personal makeover
   Give yourself a facial, or invite a professional
   Give yourself a manicure and pedicure, or invite a professional
   Meditate, chant, and sing
   Record your voice, listen back to it, and explore your tones
      and inflections
   Study acupressure and apply to yourself

Talk to yourself in a mirror and explore how others see you
Develop your speaking and presentation skills, then video-
   tape

Laptop Projects

Being on bed rest compelled me to finally buy a laptop. Laptops are so much more manageable for your bed or chair environment than trying to use a desktop computer. For instance, a laptop fits well on an able table or lap tray.

Once you are connected to a computer or laptop, your opportunities are virtually limitless. I would subscribe to Skype and Netflix immediately, and to the *New York Times* digital delivery for your personal areas of interest (health, style, business, politics, international news, etc.).

With access to the Internet, you can download everything you've ever wanted to know about any subject: medicine, sports, travel, art history, politics, human anatomy, herbal remedies, gemstones—it is all there. You can join chat sessions with your friends, associates, local news reporters, and physicians.

The best way to become acquainted with what is available is to start asking via Google. Start searching and familiarize yourself with the Google universe. Exploring topics online will keep you busy for as long as you remain interested.

The time spent on the Internet costs money depending on your contract with your Internet service provider (ISP). You should find a provider that offers a monthly plan that suits your budget and anticipated time on line. Depending on your plan, remember to disconnect after use; otherwise, you will be charged for the time.

There is an ocean of software on almost any subject matter, available to you by downloading right onto your computer. Learning and exploring online is invigorating. Tutorials on anything will enrich your knowledge and life experience, on and off bed rest! For example, Photoshop, Illustrator and iPhoto are wonderful programs for advanced creative exploration.

Computer Encouragement

Computers are educational, interactive, creative, and offer something for every-one. They are the best way to connect with loved ones and associates, be interac-tive and creative, while extending yourself far beyond immobility. Additionally, you can connect with millions of others who are physically confined and share information, especially about the latest innovations or personal projects.

It may seem like everyone in the world is computer savvy. If you are intimi-dated by computers, now is the time to learn and explore more, in a low pressure setting.

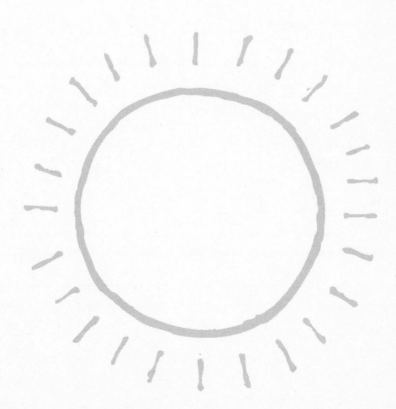

CHAPTER NINE

YOU'RE NOT ALONE

Everyone who experiences extended physical confinement, either through strict bed rest or being immobilized, has their own unique journey trying to cope. As you will see by the following stories, there is a common thread among them: a positive desire to make the most of the challenge. You are not alone!

Susan, 39 years old, "The faith to carry on."

My bed rest experience occurred in the heart of winter. Frequent snow cover added a silence and stillness that conveniently supported my situation. The weather and time of year helped me relax into a cocoon of calm, but so did important people in my life. My initial reaction to being put on bed rest for preterm labor was outrage, and a shock to my system. I had planned to be one of those pregnant ladies who exercised right through my pregnancy to the day I delivered. I had been accustomed to running, cycling, swimming in lakes, and cross-country skiing on a regular basis. I worked in an art studio and was on my feet all day, teaching graduate students and artists in the community how to tackle oversized stretched canvases for large paintings.

Unexpectedly, I was unable to walk to the toilet without contractions, which sent me to the hospital two days prior for intensive obstetric care and observation. I was in preterm labor and sentenced to bed rest for the remainder of my pregnancy. I went deep within for a new kind of strength to endure this unexpected hardship, and at the same time my husband looked to me for how he could help. His warm and supportive ways were invaluable, and his reassurance became my wellspring of hope and patience. He encouraged me to accept the conditions for the sake of the baby's and my health, and to do everything to settle comfortably into our new reality. He assured me he would manage our every need, and he did so by cooking, cleaning, shopping, communicating with others, and doing everything that needed attention! He had a good sense of humor on top of this big upset, and he showered me with loving gestures, drawing a not-too-hot but not-too-cold bath for me, fluffing pillows, massaging my shoulders, and frequent kisses! Others in our family and small community also helped me with small but meaningful "gifts" such as superb book recommendations, and short but wonderful visits with bags of groceries and precooked meals. I figured out my own helpful treatments: two Tylenol in the morning, two cups of water every hour, and two ultralight exercise sessions a day (limited isometrics approved by my ob-gyn).

I tried to keep to a daily schedule that included reading the morning paper, eating a delicious breakfast prepared by my husband, light yoga after breakfast (only my face, neck, feet, and arms), and making phone calls before eating my lunch. As I settled calmly into acceptance, bed rest was peaceful, productive, and actually enjoyable.

I ate only for nutritional reasons. I preferred small quantities of food, and I sat up to aid my digestion. I wasn't worried about gaining weight, but I definitely did not want to feel heavy from eating the wrong foods. I ate soup and salad, yogurt and fruit, small pieces of bread and crackers, and a little bit of chocolate. I liked feeling agile, regardless of the fact that I could hardly move, especially compared to my normal levels of activity. In retrospect, I probably should have sought out more massage but I wasn't certain how my body would react. My husband and I cuddled closely at night; we missed our sexual intimacy but we had no choice—we were told to refrain, as it would stimulate contractions.

I am very grateful that everything worked out successfully, and that for three months I held onto courage and faith to carry on.

Hannah, 44 years old, "You promise to help, I promise to deal!"

At just about the three-mile mark, the farthest point from my house, I tripped on the uneven sidewalk and fell, breaking both of my arms. It was fast; I went down face-first and tried to catch the fall with my arms. In seconds, I knew I had broken both—the sound and painful sensation were unmistakable. I still don't know how I got myself off the ground but I did, and I went immediately to the closest house on the street. Yes, something was truly not okay because I couldn't knock at the front door. So I kicked it with my foot, and by now my hands and arms were throbbing. I'm a nurse, and I realized that I was just short of going into shock.

An elderly man opened the door, and it was my lucky day that he was nice and knew exactly why I was there without needing much conversation. He asked immediately if I had hit my head? He asked my name, my age, and what had happened? This was all so he could best help me, by calling 911 or taking me back home.

Well, I'll never forget this helpful man. He taught me exactly how to be if someone ever shows up in my life, hurt. After the big event, my husband and I brought him a gift basket. For the next eight weeks, I walked (carefully) but had no use of my arms. They were each cast up to my shoulder, and I could not feed or wipe myself, insert tampons, brush my teeth or hair, hold a phone, write, put on clothing, tie shoes, or drive.

My husband did everything for me, and we fell madly in love, to a whole new level in our twenty-two years of marriage! We laughed, we kissed, and we loved the exploration life presented.

Kimberly, 36 years old, "Where there's a will, there's a way."

Eleven years ago I was bedridden with my first pregnancy. After eight days of trying to stop labor, Alex was born at twenty-eight-weeks gestation. He weighed only two pounds, and because of complications, he spent the next seven months in the intensive care unit. I was no longer bedridden when he was born, but I was confined to the pediatric intensive care unit at the hospital, right by his side. While he grew to become strong and healthy, he was left with a lifetime disability, mild cerebral palsy. During my next pregnancy, I was extremely cautious, as I had preeclampsia, but my second boy was born without trauma, albeit two weeks early. With my third pregnancy I went into preterm labor four months before my due date, and spent the rest of the pregnancy on strict bed rest. Faced again with the possibility of a premature birth, I fully accepted the bed rest protocol.

My mother came immediately to help us, until we found some live-in help. At the time, my second son, Ben, was four years old and had just started kindergarten, and Alex was seven years old, in third grade with special needs and requirements. My mother's around-the-clock assistance was invaluable to me. We hired extra help for cleaning, cooking, and driving.

In addition, friends and neighbors were incredible! Food arrived at our home every night. Dinner deliveries continued through the first month after the new baby's birth. People knew exactly what we loved, and everything was labeled and placed in the refrigerator: green salad, main course, bread and butter, and dessert. Often, there were extra treats thrown in, such as fruits and cheeses, granolas, and chocolates. We got to the point where we had too much food and not enough space in the freezer or cupboards. One of my friends took over the scheduling and arranged for a more spread-out schedule: deliveries on Mondays, Wednesdays, and Fridays.

Neighbors volunteered to take the two boys to school, and me to doctors' appointments. They dropped off special treats throughout the days including books and new release DVDs. When the house was quiet because everyone was at school or work, I enjoyed quietly listening to National Public Radio. I brought myself up-to-date with current events and politics, a great escape from reality. I even got involved with some of the talk shows, commenting on-air about certain controversial issues. It gave me a sense of purpose far beyond the bed that I never left.

A friend who lived across the street was also pregnant. She wanted to learn how to knit, so at least twice a week, I helped her with her knitting while we talked.

Having a kindergartner meant I had "company" every afternoon. Ben would arrive home and before his nap, he would climb into bed with me. We'd read and play quiet games. When Alex arrived home later, he would do the same thing, and often the three of us would cuddle in bed, read together, play board games, or just talk. None of this might have happened so smoothly had it not been for my confinement. Small children have the capacity to understand human challenges.

I tried very hard to manage the day-to-day family needs and activities from the bed. I feared that bed rest would invite unwelcome problems for my husband and children, therefore, I tried to keep myself strong and involved. It also kept me from focusing on inevitable fear, frustration, and discomfort. To stay as sane as possible, I kept myself stimulated with news and information; I listened to podcasts on a variety of interests; I read spiritual books; and I studied Italian. When my children showed their own frustration with my limitations, we talked about it in simple terms, and I allowed them to stay home with me if that helped so they could feel close to me, and extra "attended" to. My husband had his own needs and I tried very hard to be a good partner regardless of being so limited. I believe my bed rest experience was just as hard on my family as it was on me, just in another way. We all grew and thrived in trying to make the best of the conditions every day.

Owen, 41 years old, "With a sense of humor, anything is possible."
Ever since the early sixties, when I first discovered serious cycling, I dreamed of making a pilgrimage to Europe. This was the world epicenter of the sport, the

place with the most races, the highest standards, and the greatest public specta-torship.

Unfortunately, a season in Europe was no idle financial enterprise. It took me half a decade of savings before I was able to finally go, and that was in 1972.

I lived with three other Americans in a flat near Grenoble, France, bought a used car and we were soon into the swing of the bike life. It was my dream life: eat, sleep, and ride. Like monks in the nearby monastery of the Grande Chartreuse, we lived a focused life that demanded a balance of effort and recovery. However, sometimes we left before dawn to drive to a race, rode all day in freezing rain and even snow, and returned at night to a cold dinner and even colder shower.

These and other stresses notwithstanding, I felt fit and ready for any adver-sity. One night in late June we rode a nighttime criterium under the street lights of Chambéry. As usual the rain was lashing down, but by now we were inured to its effects. One of the riders had a lapse of attention, his bike slid out from under him, and it was my misfortune to be directly behind. I hit the downed rider and was catapulted through the air onto my back with a resounding whack. It was at this point that my focus abruptly shifted from the idealized cycling life to hell in bed.

Once I was cleared from the course and my buddies found me shivering on the sidelines, they did their best to get me back to the apartment and into my bed. They laid me out, wished me well, and rushed off to eat, clean up, and get ready for the next day's outing. The ensuing quiet let me take stock of things.

The pain was located in my lower back just left of center. My father had complained of similar pains, something about his sacroiliac, and I wondered if there was a relationship. If so, then I knew nothing was broken, that somehow a nerve was pinched and I would be okay. This self-diagnosis was only a minor relief because the pain was beyond anything I had ever experienced.

I wanted to take off my clothing and crawl under the covers but the least bit of movement ignited shocks. Over the next two hours I finally got my jacket off; I gave up on the rest. By grabbing the blanket and rolling one way then back across the other way, I was finally able to get between the sheets. I stayed there for the next twenty-four hours until I was overwhelmed by the increasing urge to pee and having no clue how to get out of bed. Then I spied my water glass. Oh sweet salvation! I threw what little was left out the open window next to the bed and then filled the glass almost to the top. This, too, went out the window and down eight stories. I hoped no one below was leaning out and wondering where this urine downpour was coming from.

I had never felt so bewildered or trapped. If I lay just right, the pain was more threatening than actual. I could do absolutely nothing.

Boring! Trapped! Painful! That was the understatement for what this was, and how I felt with this crushing new reality. The hours dragged by and sometime after dark on the second day of lying there, the guys returned. They were good enough to sit around for a while, give me a description of the race results and their personal adventures, get me some food, and carry me to the bathroom. They got my water bottle off my bike so I could have my own water supply. They also piled a stack of French bike magazines next to me, the only reading material in the house. They were in France for the same reason I was, so I was on my own while they rode all day, every day.

The constant low-grade pain that would erupt into electric shock feelings at the slightest wrong move was a serious issue. But I was accustomed to adversity, like every bikie is. But there is suffering and there is suffering, and the boredom soon came to weigh on me far more than the pain. My French was still rudimentary, so the magazines were mostly valuable for the pictures. I had language books and studied them several times a day and went to great lengths to decipher passages in the magazines, but I longed for some easy and entertaining reading. There was no one to phone, and no phone to use. No TV, just endless gray skies.

I was familiar with the Zen idea of thinking about nothing, trying not to try. I remembered a psychology article I'd read some time back about the benefits of going mad. At the time the reality necessary for that was so far from my own I'd only dimly grasped the article's meaning, but now it was making more sense every day. If you could, in your mind, make a complete break with the world and enter a nicer space of your own creation, a whole order of difficulty could be resolved. I wasn't quite ready for that yet, but contemplating its attractive possibilities was no longer a vision dimly perceived, instead it was now a potential solution lurking on the other side of the bed.

Beyond boredom and pain was frustration. I was very familiar with Victor Frankl's admonition in his famous book, *Man's Search for Meaning*, which says that our ultimate freedom lies in our ability to choose our attitude toward any situation. I played with this idea a lot. I tried it out in my head. I had time to argue it and agree with it. But I came to realize it was up to me to make the most of the time while I was injured, and it didn't matter where I was—geographically or in my expectations of athletics. I was in the moment, and would be in this state for the next several weeks. Now I could really learn French, now I could really discover myself through meditation, now I could put cycling into its proper role as only a part of my life. Now I could write letters, and in fact try to resolve long-standing misunderstandings with members of my family, or at least apologize for some problems I caused in the past.

Thankfully there was a view from the room. Meditating on the interplay of the mountains and weather provided not only a form of sweet entertainment but also the inner peace I found.

After three weeks I got a surprise visit from the uncle of a French bikie who knew there had been four of us Americans and had inquired as to why there were now only three. When told, the old man came by and pushed and prodded my back and slapped on a heat plaster laced with "phenalgon," a cream derived from an extract of marmot liver and so hot that if you rubbed yourself all over, you could, I'm sure, run naked in the Arctic with impunity.

Whatever he did, it changed something, and the next day I took my first halting steps to the bathroom. In two more days I went outside and in a week I was able to get back on the salvation machine, my bike, although it was another month before I got back to the races. I was mentally stronger than ever before. I had just proven to myself that I had depths I didn't know about. I had just spent the heart of the summer discovering a new form of long "mountain climbing." It sure felt good to transfer the iron will back to the bike.

Amy, 40 years old, "Embracing the possible, amid impossible conditions."

Once I understood that staying off my feet prevented early contractions, I succumbed to doctor's orders, a fully reclined position. I chose *not* to stress, and to make the most of doing "nothing." I kept myself as healthy as I could while depending on others for shopping for good food and providing satisfying meals, and staying hydrated. I monitored my blood pressure and visualized taking this pregnancy to full term. I reminded myself hourly that this event was a three-month time-out, and that there was a lot of life to come. The inconvenience of bed rest is minor compared to the heartache of untold complications requiring long stays in the hospital. Therefore, my ability to be patient, embrace the possibilities, and accept bed rest was easy. Toward the end of my term, my doctor announced that I could get up from bed rest. I didn't. What was another two weeks to guarantee a healthy and risk-free birth!

Larry, 45 years old, "Acceptance invites opportunity, including happiness."

My lifetime career in law enforcement ended one day four years ago after a routine physical. The doctor found extensive cancer in my pancreas. There was no choice but to agree to immediate surgery, previously one of my greatest fears.

My story is somewhat of a miracle. I have healed and resumed a normal life, yet I never would have guessed the power of the mind and spirit had I not lain quietly for four months on bed rest. Reflecting back, it was the potency of family love, friendships, and my own self-discovery that pulled me through, especially the many hours, days, and weeks of quietude. Bed rest afforded me the time to empower myself. The love from family and friends, the feeling of accomplishment and overall pleasure from activities that brought me deep personal joy, opened the way for successful healing.

Prior to this experience, I was not a big communicator. I did not spend time with myself in any significant way except to be physically present as a father, husband, and law officer. While I had a lot going on in my head, it usually churned away inside of me and spilled out at work: at meetings, training sessions, etc. From the time I learned of my illness through the early days of recovery, there was a significant personal shift. For the first time in my life, I became aware of my inner self; I began reaching out, sharing, and expressing myself. In turn, I was showered with the deepest love a man can know. Through stillness and self-discovery, I grew stronger and healthier.

A profound revelation from my bed rest experience is that every individual has the ability to go way beyond his or her status quo. Prior to my bed rest experience, I was not in touch with certain interests, personal feelings, and other aspects of my whole self. I spent little or no time thinking about the meaning of relationships or the value of love. I have always been very practical and lived my life with structure and ambition. For instance, I had no idea who I really was deep inside. I didn't know I was capable of true feelings and spiritual thoughts. My experience on bed rest was a gift in that it opened up another dimension of who I am. Now, I'm a bigger person, and I experience more from everyday interactions and activity than I ever have before. I learned something very important about all people. Whether you're old or young, in school or at work, on a soccer field or in bed for months, there is a whole other level of potential within ready to be tapped.

Margaret, 48 years old, "There's a silver lining behind every dark cloud."

When I was in my late twenties, my podiatrist recommended foot surgery for a problem that had been bothering me for almost a decade. I was virtually crippled by this time: walking was painful, and running was almost impossible. The bunions on my feet had become so large and arthritic, I could only wear shoes if I cut holes in the front corners. My afternoons spent running seven to ten miles were over. I couldn't find peace of mind or body due to the incessant pain. I decided to have the surgery, and given my healthy, independent, and resourceful ways, I imagined that I would bounce back immediately.

That was not the script. I was bedridden for six weeks. I was completely unprepared, and forced to depend on others for personal and domestic care. In the meantime, I could crawl, but after one afternoon of it, I succumbed to staying in bed.

As hard as it was for me to embrace my new reality, I did, and I suddenly had contact with people, and enjoyed it! I realized, perhaps for the first time in my life, how important human connections are, and that helping others is important, as is receiving help from others. It is often said that we learn life lessons the hard way, and this was the case for me right now.

My feet finally healed, the bunions are history, and I am back to walking, running, and living my active and independent existence. Yet now I look to help others in need, and also to open myself to receiving help when I have needs. The quiet time in bed was a special gift as well as an important lesson.

Ginger, 38 years old, "A small price to pay for a life-long reward."

I was first diagnosed as a DES daughter when I was seventeen (the result of the synthetic estrogen drug diethylstilbestrol). I was told at the time that I had a "hood" on my cervix (that was later cauterized off), but that there were no other symptoms of DES exposure that I should be concerned about, especially with regards to pregnancy.

My husband and I learned about our first pregnancy in January 1986. I was twenty-eight. When my physician confirmed the pregnancy, our hopes and dreams began. On my third prenatal visit, one of the older members of the ob-gyn team examined me for the first time and asked me if I had been pregnant before. I said no. His response to me was, "Well, you had better chalk this pregnancy up to history, as you will never carry this baby to term. You don't have a cervix that is worth mentioning." I was devastated and very frightened. I went home and searched for another doctor. The second ob-gyn was very supportive and told me to take it easy, no vacuuming or lifting, and that it would probably be a good idea not to have any sex while pregnant.

We carried on in a fragile state for the next couple of months. I quit my job and "hung around the house." I couldn't wait to go out and buy my first maternity outfit. Ironically, the day that I bought my first maternity dress was the day that my cervix started to dilate. It was mid-May and I had seven more months to be pregnant. The doctor put me on bed rest immediately and said to keep my feet higher than my heart. I stayed that way for six days until my next appointment when it was decided that I needed to go to a perinatal specialist. Upon my arrival, I went into labor. I was rushed to the local hospital and put in a Trendelenburg position, a bed position where the head is kept lower than the feet. At this point my doctor decided that a vaginal cerclage, a stitch sewn to keep the cervix closed, wouldn't hold, and they began thinking about an abdominal cerclage. I was then pumped full of drugs—terbutaline was the main one—and given a bedpan. I remember thinking, "How is this going to work if I am on my head?"

The labor stopped, thanks to the drugs, and luckily they let me put the bed in a normal position for my toilet needs. I ate and slept and received visitors in the Trendelenburg position for the next four weeks. The hospital became my safe haven and I felt peaceful and hopeful. My mother, who lived on the other side of the country, put her life on hold, and stayed by my bed from sunup to sundown each and every day. It was an incredible time for the two of us; after all she had taken the drug DES to save her pregnancy, which in turn had put my pregnancy in danger. Now I was taking any drug they gave me to save my baby.

After five weeks, it was decided that I could return home and await the arrival of the baby. The second day home, I began leaking amniotic fluid, which was not a good sign. I knew the baby was only twenty-five weeks at best. Back to the hospital we went, straight to my old room, which was still available. In all honesty, I felt relieved to be back on my head, and safe. Four days later my water broke. We were at twenty-seven weeks, our big goal, and we achieved it. My doctor announced that there was going to be a birthday, he was ready to let me give birth. My family, friends, and I were thrilled, and there was true joy on all of our faces. The staff did an incredible job of "playing along" with the happy occasion, never letting on that they knew what a twenty-seven-week-old baby meant. We delivered a two-pound, five-ounce son by C-section, and immediately felt the incredible joy of parenthood.

Our perception continued to be that we had delivered a perfectly healthy baby. They had said two pounds was good; we gave them two pounds, five ounces! They said twenty-six weeks was good, we gave them twenty-seven! Within the hour we were told that the baby's lungs had collapsed and that he had a hemorrhage on his brain. It was only a short time later that a doctor I did not know walked in, looked at Jim and me, and said the words that I will never forget, "Your baby has died."

My friends at the hospital taught us how to deal with the grief. We slowly returned to "real life" and began making plans for our next baby. We scheduled our next surgery for the abdominal cerclage the following January. It was felt that performing the surgery in a non-pregnant state might give the doctors a better chance of placing the cerclage in a more secure way. Abdominal cerclages were supposed to be a one-time surgery. My previous one had ruptured and had to be removed during the C-section.

I found out I was pregnant again in August of that year, 1987. I was incredibly calm about this second pregnancy and had a gut feeling that we were going to be OK. The doctors were very cautious in their care, and kept making reference to the fact that we now had a "history." I was put on strict bed rest at approximately eighteen weeks. My doctor told me that bed rest meant only getting up to go to the bathroom. I begged for a shower a day if I promised to sit down during the shower. The medical team gave me that gift. I remember buying a small stool because it was wide enough to be comfortable. My mother-in-law came from Vermont and moved in with us for the last three months of the pregnancy. I remember feeling very Zen about this time on bed rest. I initially thought about learning a new language, books I wanted to read, old movies I wanted to see, etc. The most memorable experiences from that bed rest time were the visits from friends who would bring lunch and their Scrabble board or a movie. I couldn't read because my mind simply wandered, and I spent hours looking up at the ceiling while counting knotholes. I didn't watch television. I didn't knit or learn a foreign language either. My only attention seemed to be on making that baby. I do remember wishing a couple of times that my mother-in-law would fly back to Vermont!

We set up a queen-size mattress in the living room. In the morning I would shower, dress, eat, and move to the living room before my husband went to work. I didn't return to the bedroom until it was time to go to bed. I found this to be crucial to my mental health, and it also helped my husband and my mother-in-law as well. Peace of mind came from my use of a Tokos home monitor. This device read my uterine activity for two one-hour sessions a day. A nurse would call and ask me to send the information over the phone lines. They would read the strips and let me know if I had any activity. Whenever I felt nervous or unsure about my activity, I could put the monitor on and call in my strip, anytime of night or day. This was a great way to keep my stress level from getting too high. The one time when the strip was overly active, I was told to lie on my left side and drink a lot of water. The daily contact with the staff at Tokos was imperative to my daily routine. They were just a phone call away.

We didn't have any "hairy" moments during this pregnancy. At thirty-seven weeks, I began to have some pain at the site of the cerclage that was reminiscent of my previous pain when my cerclage was rupturing. I phoned the specialist who advised I come down right away. Some urgency returned as I could not go into labor yet because of the cerclage and the vertical incision that had been made in my uterus when I delivered James Peter, our first son who had died.

My daughter Chalen was born at thirty-seven weeks. She was six pounds, nine ounces, nineteen inches long. The cerclage had ruptured and had to be removed again. Chalen was truly my miracle baby.

We ended up moving back to Vermont four years later. I had just finished graduate school and was hired as a speech-language pathologist in Stowe, Vermont. Chalen, Jim, and I were getting used to a new life when we discovered that we were pregnant again. This was a total surprise, as we were just getting used to the idea of having only one child. I was petrified. I had just taken a new job, and I knew what my pregnancies entailed. I immediately called my perinatologist in California. I needed to know if I was tempting fate by asking for another child. His answer was no.

We began the process again. I went in for surgery at twelve weeks for my third cerclage. The surgery was a success and I recovered well and went back to work for four weeks before being placed once again on strict bed rest. We were a little smarter this time, and I realized that I needed to be "organized" while juggling bed rest and motherhood. I determined that I needed not to do this all alone, and I asked for help, other than from family. I hired a housecleaner to come in and do the kitchen and bathroom. I had a mattress company deliver a firm foam mattress for the den, and a body pillow. The medical team set up the Tokos program, not without a slight argument, but I won! I needed peace of mind. We set up two moveable trays—one for daytime items, one for night creams, medications, and water bottles. We stationed me centrally in the house, where I could see the front door from my bed as well as out the large living room window with a view.

I started hooking a Persian-style rug, which helped pass the time. I read a lot of books to my daughter, a very bonding time. We got satellite television, which meant that I could watch all the old movies I missed the other times on bed rest. We already had a success story, so we were confident that now was a matter of trying to pass the time.

I moved around the house a little more, but lifted absolutely nothing. We rented a nice leather recliner for the living room instead of being on a mattress. It was better for having visitors; it made everyone feel more comfortable.

At thirty-six weeks, I began to feel the twinges of labor. We called the doctors, and they said to come in for an ultrasound. Our son Peter was born five hours later, six pounds, nine ounces, nineteen inches long (exactly the same as his sister!).

There isn't a day that goes by that I don't look at my children and think about how lucky I am to have them! I look back on the bed rest experiences with mixed feelings. I miss the structure of those days. I always knew what to expect. It was more positive than negative because of what bed rest meant for my health and the future of our family life. It's a small price to pay for such an incredible outcome.

Yvette, 36 years old, "Being positive is life's sunshine no matter the weather."

An exciting midmorning visit to my ob-gyn for a seven-month pregnancy check changed not only our much anticipated vacation plans, but our family's life for one entire summer. My husband and I had been looking forward to taking a special vacation for a much-needed break from our busy lives and to celebrate our dream of having a child together. We had our family life with my daughter from another marriage, six years old and very much the center of every day. Gideon and I had been trying to get pregnant for four out of the five years we were married. Unfortunately, I had been struggling with chronic fatigue syndrome, and our chances for success looked slim. Now we were so happy and I hadn't felt this good in over a year!

The baby had dropped so low and moved into position so prematurely that it put tremendous pressure on my lower organs and back. My doctor feared the blood supply to the placenta would be impacted by this position and that premature labor might be a possibility. I experienced early contractions at six months and had severe sciatica during the fourth and fifth months. Whether the doctor had ordered bed rest or not, I would have put myself on it. My legs and hips felt locked around my tight and enormous uterus. There was no question my body needed to be reclined.

My husband was fantastic. He saw the writing on the wall as far as the limitations, and immediately took on multiple roles.

We were not in a financial position to hire someone to stay with me, so Gideon approached everyone at his office to explain the bed rest predicament, and quickly transferred his normal office to a home office. Throughout my two months on bed rest, he did all the cooking, carpooling, dishes, etc. We did hire someone to come in once a week to do general cleaning and laundry.

Luckily, being confined to bed did not present a problem for my work, since I'm a teacher and I had just finished the school year. However, I had looked forward to spending quality time with my daughter during these summer months, since afterwards there would be an addition to the family and inevitable changes.

I never really had a routine while on bed rest. It was summer so there was less pressure and no time constraints. My daughter took it upon herself to set up a chair right next to the places where I rested: the couch, the outdoor cot, my bed, or the reclined chair in the living room. There she would sit, and either read to me or have me read to her. Nothing held us back from traveling around the house to eat, talk, and read together. In my bedridden state, I felt a little bit like a bird moving from one tree perch to another. After hours of lying in one spot, it felt good to move on to the next place.

I spent a lot of time talking with friends on the telephone. Many fellow teachers and neighbors called to cheer me up although I was truly in good spirits because I was preparing to give birth. I read many magazines, and I listened to music more than usual. My daughter's portable piano allowed us to practice scales together and encouraged us to keep up our practice. We also had paints and blank canvases so our artistic ways were encouraged. My daughter and I created some beautiful collaborations, which are framed and hung in our new home. My favorite activity was knitting a colorful blanket for the baby while my daughter knit doll blankets right next to me.

I missed sexual intimacy with Gideon; however, we did a lot of cuddling. Gideon gave me back massages and loved to rub my belly. I will never forget this part of my bed rest or how relaxing, simple, and special this quiet phase truly was for me, and our family.

Holly, 46 years old, "Warm your heart with a spot of sunshine or a cup of tea!"

I had gestational diabetes and other preterm labor complications, and given my age, there was no arguing that I should be bedridden for the duration of my pregnancy, three months of stillness. I worked from my bed but not without reducing my full time hours by half. I had to be still, and also to focus on a whole new diet that was very restricted and regimented. My doctor discovered gestational diabetes during my standard prenatal glucose test. For the next three months I had to draw blood from my fingers four times a day, and also moderate my glucose level. Daily, I took a urine sample to check for ketones, a type of insulin analysis. I also kept a diary of everything I ate, drank, chewed, and swallowed. I could only consume high-protein foods and carbohydrates. No sweets, which meant giving up my big pregnancy craving, a Snapple. Mostly I ate chicken, fish, cheese, and vegetables. The new dietary guide involved three snacks in addition to regular meals, which was new for me. I was willing to do anything to stay healthy, for the dream baby and me. My husband's words of encouragement helped so much; he would always say, "This kind of diet will surely produce an exceptionally beautiful baby!"

I drank a lot of tea. Not only was it important for me to keep up my liquids, it was cold not moving and staying put in our shady home. I tried to make the best of the conditions because it wasn't going to do anybody any good to panic over my lying in bed. Fresh air breezing through the windows reminded me to stay positive. I also moved to different places, following the sun as it moved across the sky and shined from room to room. I found myself falling asleep on a mattress or chair in all sorts of sunny spots, like a mother cat. This truly helped my moods and the passing of time.

Perrin, 36 years old, "It takes a village!"

It was a hot Labor Day weekend. I was twenty-six weeks pregnant with my third child and I began bleeding at the neighborhood picnic. When I called my doctor, he wasn't sure wha was occurring but thought that there might be a tear or hole in the placenta during the amniocentesis. Nothing definite would be known until delivery.

When we arrived at the hospital within an hour of the call, he was there, too, and it didn't take long to be informed that I wouldn't return home for ten weeks, not until the new baby arrived. My husband and two children turned white, and in my mind, there was no time for drama. Not now, I had to get on the phone to get help at home!

I had had four pregnancies prior to this one. Two were miscarriages, and two were golden—our two beautiful children now age four and six. Oh, I treasure them, and I did not want to be separated.

I called a dear friend, a woman who felt like my great aunt, who agreed to take over the first week. After we all adjusted, my mother arrived to help lighten the load for Mary who stayed on as our primary day caregiver, a lifesaver! The plan was that she would stay with us part time until the baby arrived. My sister planned to arrive during the fourth week and various people would follow.

Home life hummed along and everyone adapted, learned to become more self-sufficient, and accepted that life wasn't ideal, especially for "Mom" stuck in the hospital. Our friends and neighbors sent meals to the house, they organized carpools for the kids, and one family even loaned us their automatic car so that grandma could drive.

I spent much of my time reading, enjoying the newspaper, and watching the news. I hadn't had this much quiet or focused time in years. I finished craft projects such as a cross-stitch pillow for the baby and two hand-knit sweaters for each of my kids. I continued with as much of the volunteer work as I usually did; they sent me letters and envelopes to stuff and I made some fundraising phone calls during a pledge drive.

The hospital staff was fantastic. I really enjoyed getting to know the nurses and obstetrical students who interviewed me while the doctor examined me. Everyone seemed to read my mind just when I found a new concern. For instance, I was worried about losing muscle strength; it was a long time being completely immobile. A physical therapist arrived immediately to show me some upper body exercises with an elastic band. She encouraged the nurses to give me a body massage when they came in to check me—the arms, feet, and neck! I missed being physical, as much as I missed being outdoors. That fall was the most beautiful weather (I could see a little from my window). The nurses and my family decided to wheel me outdoors, and twice my husband and the kids wheeled me to a park near the hospital! Everyone helped me to make the most of my bed rest.

One rather private but important matter: I missed the sexual intimacy with my husband, and I know he missed this, too.

The staff neonatologist, who visited occasionally, helped me to realize I was doing the smart thing by being in the hospital for immediate response should anything occur. The possibility of hemorrhaging was high, and it would be foolish to risk the baby's or my life.

I delivered a daughter, Abby, two pounds, nine ounces, at thirty-one-and-a-half weeks. What a time this was, but in the overall scope of a long and healthy life, it was a short test and exercise with patience. All for a very worthwhile cause.

Darcy, 41 years old, "Long-term bed rest is like hiking Mt. Everest. Trekking is the time spent healing, reaching the summit is complete recovery, life-changing."

I am a doctor who completed four years of bed rest. My husband and I, our six-year-old son and four-and-a-half-year-old daughter took a trip to San Diego, and I was feeling some back pain when we returned. But I had to be tough, and get right back to the hospital and my patients. My back became so painful that I considered calling a physical therapist; in the meantime I took pain relief meds. I worked day and night, as doctor and mother, with constant twinges in my back. About three weeks into it, I was alone with the kids one afternoon and in an effort to calm my daughter during a tantrum, I attempted to pick her up but she resisted, and so did my back. In the back of my mind, I was very concerned. Could I truly continue with patients? No. From then on, it's been four years of treatment, numerous surgeries, and bed rest recovery.

The worst part of this injury was that I could not sit. If that had been possible, I would have been "mobile" in a wheelchair, at least I could be wheeled around and go places. Or I could have used a motorized cart, go places in the car. It took five months before a back specialist made the diagnosis of internal disk disruption. And, because two disks were involved, there was initially little likelihood of help from surgery. The recommendation we decided to try was to simulate the surgery situation, which was to immobilize my spine by fusion. The surgeon recommended a body cast, and I agreed. The cast went from above my breast all the way down to mid-thigh, immobilizing the hip joint completely. Initially, it was very traumatic because I couldn't keep up with my personal hygiene. No one had prepared me for what accessories would be required with the body cast. Now there are endless resources and ways to get beyond such extreme immobility, but I was a pioneer, and while this was initially overwhelming, my husband (also a doctor) and some friends discovered solutions.

There were more surgeries, month-long hospital stays, and complications, and bed rest became my existence. The thoughts of working again, future vacations, and the unending child care and housecleaning expenses were grim. I developed benign vertigo because of the immobilization. I was told that this happens from not exercising and being in one position for too long. My heart rate also went up; my doctor said I had Astronaut Syndrome, because I was always lying down without any exertion stress on my body. I had another surgery that went well and by the time I left the hospital, I was walking for half-hour stretches and making my way up and down stairs. There wasn't a twinge in my body! I felt great!

Upon returning home, I felt the urge simply to cut back the pain medicine since I didn't have pain. I found a physical therapist who focused on my shoulders, and started light core- and leg-strengthening exercises. In addition, I hired a Feldenkrais therapist who came twice a week. I was *committed* to doing everything to get me whole again. Using my body and having hands work on my body made me feel so much better. The power of touch is phenomenal.

Physical therapy in conjunction with a vitamin management regime was key to continued recovery. It got me out of bed and over time made strength and healing continue.

One practice that we have all adopted since my injury is hydration and wise nutrition. We eat simply—fruit and veggies, and gluten-free for ease of digestion. We refrain from sweets and meats. Smart eating is key to being energized and positive, and healthy for life. Today, I am stronger and more involved in our family life than ever before. The spirit of our family has also healed; everyone is happy.

There continue to be positive aspects of my bed rest experience. While I miss practicing medicine, I am well networked in our community, all through social media. I manage two soccer teams and teach the parents how to use their computers for all communication. The kids and I shop for clothes online, rather than driving around and spending our valuable time looking around. When it's time for piano lessons, we all learn from the same teachers. I taught myself on an electric keyboard while bedridden, and the kids learned, too. We have all grown in special ways. I believe our family meetings over the months and years, which were open and sensitive, have set the stage for two strong and capable young people who carry deep compassion and the capability to help others. Bed rest was a gift in many ways.

My approach to being physically confined was not always so positive. But I realized, while in suffer-mode, that one either sinks or swims while enduring a situation like mine. I made the choice to come to terms with it, even while adjusting to a completely new identity. I used to feel very sorry for myself, which caused isolation. With acceptance, I got better, climbed a big mountain in Life, saw the view, and now have a whole new perspective in living fully every day.

I would never have made it without a few key discoveries: wearing a watch and labeling the medicine vial(s) on the side and top. The wedge pillow was a great source of physical comfort. Earplugs were essential. My "grab it stick" allowed me to pick up paper, pencils, and other small things. A bluetooth allowed me to use my hands while talking on the phone, and reduced tension in my neck and shoulders. Remote controls for lights and the TV help with independence. The other items I used on bed rest:

Massage table—for the field trips or outings that can't be missed

Commode—portable non-flush toilet if bathroom is too far

Anti-bacterial wipes

Straws

Mug with family photo

Personal needs table: creams, medicine, drinks, note cards, tissue

Your own set of house keys to drop out of the window down to someone in the case of an emergency

Makeup with mirror—I've had fun with this for myself and with my daughter
Electric toothbrush—eliminates the arm motion/body motion
Small pet for having company: fish, cat, hamster, rat

Madeleine, 54 years old, "Perseverance against all odds!"

My medical problems involved an environmental illness combined with an autoimmune weakness that required periods of bed rest and very limited physical activity. For twelve years, I often felt tired, I "got sick" easily, and I had to spend long periods of time in bed resting to prevent an illness like a cold or the flu. I live in northern California, and in the winters I had reactions to the dampness and increased mold due to a lot of rain. In the summer, warm days that held air pollution and pollen invited more problematic reactions that caused me to feel exhausted and in need of rest.

My illness really frightened me. I would be so sick at times that I had to stay in bed for days. I never knew how long it would take to regain my strength from each bout of illness, and sometimes I could barely digest my food. At other times, my body ached all over. Often, I had severe respiratory problems like bronchitis. I would also be weakened by bladder infections. These are all typical symptoms associated with the syndrome called environmental illness.

I was consumed with fear until one bright sunny day when I couldn't stay in bed any longer. I summoned the physical and emotional energy I needed to get up and go outside, even though I could barely walk. My husband drove me to the Berkeley Marina, where I found a large, beautiful, sandy area. I laid on the sand and felt its warmth. There was nothing I was allergic to! I inhaled soft currents of salty air from the bay, and awakened with the cool winds from the Pacific. I felt renewed by the blue sky and the sun, and the whole mix of nature. From that moment, I was rejuvenated, and I held on to this beautiful experience. I use it as a daily reminder of what's possible with an open, positive, and energized frame of mind. I decided to travel to warm beach areas after this, and it enhanced my life exponentially! By transferring this special scenery into my bed-room, I discovered a special push to be lighter in spirit, happy, and productive. Simultaneously, I was released from my own nagging disappointment, and I felt empowered to accept this challenging phase of life. I lived with openness now, a new perspective on my illness, and new energy for the times when I couldn't get out of bed or couldn't be as productive as desired.

I thank my illness and all the time I spent resting in bed for reintroducing me to the power of nature, and for helping me to accept myself without having to prove myself through physical activity or profound accomplishments. I have attained personal peace, by learning to deeply enjoy quiet time and making the most of it—a major shift in life for someone who had at one time thrived on be-ing overly ambitious with achieving goals.

Phyllis, 57 years old, "Life happens. Keep breathing."

I woke up one morning in November literally unable to walk. It was terrifying because I had just recently recovered from hip replacement. When my surgeon x-rayed my hip, he determined I had an acute complication with the surrounding nerves, related to sciatica, and that I would have to lie on my back for at least a week icing it and resting. This would cure me.

Fortunately, my small business is headquartered at home, where I design and sew silk flowers. The upcoming Christmas season would be a busy time, and I was determined to continue to manufacture my product. So, I lay on my back and sewed for hours. With headphones in my ears, listening to music and inter-esting podcasts, I made all the flowers I needed to fill my orders, kept my sanity, and lay still long enough to resolve my ailment. I also read a great deal during this time. At one point I had my husband gather all of my large hardcover art books, and bring them to the bedside. He put together a stable table next to my bed, and I devoured each one. In two weeks, I gave myself a comprehensive art history education! When it was time to begin walking and resume an erect lifestyle, I wasn't finished with my "coursework." I breathed like I did in yoga, and carried on with normal life, including studying earnestly while feverishly catching up with everything else that had to be put on hold.

My time in bed gave me an opening to a facet of life I would have missed entirely. Who would have guessed being immobilized would be a gift!

Jason, 33 years old, "There's power in knowing that every day is one more day closer to recovery."

At the age of twenty-two, I was in a bad motorcycle accident, pinned under a truck. I sustained some serious injuries: a head concussion, a broken cheekbone, three broken ribs, and many bruises. I had severe lacerations on my leg from the under part of the vehicle, and was in the hospital in intensive care for three days. Much of the healing time was due to 180 staples put into my leg—the brake peg was lodged in my calf. Luckily, there was no permanent damage, but I just had to be still to let it heal. I was released from the hospital after a week and put on bed rest for the next month.

Television was my savior. I transferred my love of doing sports and being really fit to watching sports on TV, thank you Universal Sports! My friends visited regularly; they couldn't believe of all people that I was stuck in bed! My dad, with whom I lived, was no help at all. Too bad, because the only thing I could do alone was go to the bathroom. I needed a lot of help with getting food, water, and lots of other things you don't think about until you can't reach them. I might have starved to death but my friends didn't let that happen. They brought me water, juice, my favorite foods, magazines, and a lot of good laughs. I never dipped into depression although I could see this happening. I felt lucky to be alive. I spent a lot of my time with my headphones in, just staring into space. I worried a little bit about losing all my fitness from just lying around, but I knew once I healed, I would be back at it. I stayed positive, and knew that every day was one more day closer to getting back to normal.

Sheryl, 66 years old, "A honeymoon wrapped in stillness."

One afternoon, in the heat of the Arizona desert, I suddenly fell into my wheel-barrow. I tripped on the vines I was pruning. I fell hard, and I remember thinking how awkwardly I landed. The next thing I knew, I was lying in a hospital bed, in darkness.

I learned that my fall was serious, that I had punctured one eyeball and se-verely scratched the other on the vine's thorns. I had not been wearing sun-glasses, and it was assumed this injury would leave me blind. My husband found me unconscious, rushed me to the hospital, and surgery occurred immediately. I was left to recover in darkness and stillness for the next three to four months. Success, if any, would be found in my stillness. Any head motion would disturb the essential alignment my doctors aimed for.

I am a naturally meditative type, and the stillness required to heal served to strengthen my appreciation of being in the moment. Most people do not like to watch time pass, while I love to.

My children were grown and out of our home, and so my responsibilities to others were negligible. My husband was semi-retired and very capable and willing to prepare our meals. He had to feed me. We often drank tea together, and I listened to books on tape with my headphones, or we shared the time and listened together. These were special times, and to this day we've continued in this way (except I feed myself).

I strongly believe my accident enhanced our lives, bringing us closer, forcing us to appreciate our health, and our loyalty to one another in the face of adver-sity. The experiences we shared during this acute time took us beyond healing, to another world of spiritual oneness and joy. Our children, who came to visit many times, commented openly on the dramatic change they observed in our recharged marriage!

My sight returned after six months. My love of gardening also returned, but that took just short of a year from injury. Now, my husband gardens by my side. I believe his new interest in co-gardening is less about being worried I will fall in the wheelbarrow and more about enjoying our time together! There's a silver lining behind every dark cloud.

Jennifer, 37 years old, "There are many ways to enlightenment."

I've always fantasized about pregnancy and envisioned myself active and demonstrating that commonly talked about "glow." In my wildest dreams, I never pictured the experience I had.

Initially I'd been sentenced to rest at home on the couch or the bed for the duration of my pregnancy. I was allowed to get up to use the bathroom and fix a light lunch. The isolation in itself was a challenge. I remember bumping into a good friend in a store two days after I received these doctor's orders. She wanted to know what I was doing out of bed? I realized she was right, that my health condition had not quite sunk in, and that I was being negligent. I settled down and stayed at home from that point forward.

The holiday season was approaching. I was excited about my parents' visit, the buzz in the air, and the anticipation of my first baby! All of this kept me going during this first phase of bed rest. Then it turned cold and gray. I watched our home become messier by the day. I couldn't get up to do the things I wanted and needed to do. There was junk mail everywhere, newspapers, dirty dishes, and laundry overflowing onto the floor. I felt alone and helpless, and depressed.

My hospital bed rest came unexpectedly. A one-day trip to be monitored for contractions led to the two-and-a-half-month hospital stay. I received countless shots of terbutaline and never left the hospital again until my son was born.

The time in the hospital was one of the most emotionally trying and physically challenging times I've ever known. Without the help of the nurses, and their fantastic relaxation techniques, I might not have survived. Instead, I thrived, knowing that this was meant to support a healthy birth and baby. I was monitored for contractions around the clock. The large white belt that was constantly wrapped around my huge belly felt like an uncomfortable daily uniform. One of the nurses called me "Beautiful" and I absorbed it to turn my spirits positive. The constant sound of paper tape flowing from the monitor was nerve wracking, but with earplugs and my iPhone, I replaced it with my favorite songs! I spent hours staring at the monitor, a tall glass of water, and the helpful straw. I meditated and listened to podcasts. Friends visited and brought me delicious food. Sometimes the nurses shared parts of good films; I relied on and probably overused my Netflix account for movie rentals. Knowing my body was being fed with so much medication was hard, but I trusted my medical team and knew that this was the way to the gift of a healthy baby. One of the highlights was the nurses' massages.

Looking back, the bed rest experience was like a crash course in crisis management and self-discovery: finding ways to thrive in solitary confinement! My strength to carry on came from supportive people and creative ideas for self-preservation and happiness. I suggest if you are on bed rest, for any reason, designate helpers. If you define a job for someone to do, whether you're paying them or not, you have an agreement and there's no need to feel guilty or uncomfortable asking for help, especially when it's obvious there's a special need. People all around possess the capacity to give, and don't underestimate the incredible healing power in giving and receiving—for everyone. Friends and family can do so much to help. For someone immobilized, just be clear as to what you need!

Kendra, 35 years old, "Stillness of body opens the senses, energizing all experience."

In the spring of 1992, while traveling, I became sick with a viral illness. I expected that it would pass within a couple of weeks, but it lingered for the duration of my trip. When I returned home I no longer had the signs of acute infection in my throat, lungs, and sinuses, but other disturbing symptoms showed up. My sleep was frequently disturbed and seemed to offer no relief for the fatigue I felt during the day, which caused me to have to lie down for over half of my waking hours.

After a thorough physical exam and a lot of lab tests, the doctors found nothing to explain these disabling symptoms. Eventually, I would receive a diagnosis of chronic fatigue syndrome, but no one could ever explain what was happening at the onset or offer a cure for what ensued.

After two weeks of misery, I slipped into private despair, but not for long, as I thankfully found a way out of this darkness through the simplest embrace of self-recognition and surrender. Ten years previous to the onset of my illness, my father's unexpected death confronted me with the fact that he was suffering, and the more he pretended he wasn't, the more ill he became. I was so intrigued by this ill-fated situation, that soon after his death, I went to India to grieve and also to search for answers about physical states in illness. I inquired about spiritual struggle and the art of opening one's heart to the inevitable challenges in Life. A guru helped me understand how to stop wanting to be different, to let go of resistance, and to love in all conditions. Here I was, ten years later, in what felt like a midterm exam to see if I sufficiently learned the material!

In lying still with little physical energy, I awakened to the fact that I was suffering deeply, and not just physically. My unidentifiable symptoms in fact persisted the harder I tried to avoid the unpleasant symptoms. I found energy and light with the realization that I was immobilized for a reason, forced to take time to reflect and practice Truth. Once I surrendered, sweet peace revealed itself. Within two weeks, much of my physical pain lessened, the severe fatigue disappeared, and healthy sleep patterns returned.

Almost three years have passed since the onset of my experience of bed rest. I continue to experience some disabling fatigue and pain, and I continue to experiment with a variety of treatments to regain normalcy of health. But my intuition tells me that before long, I will be physically active and a hundred percent healthy. Yet this time has been the richest spiritually I have ever known.

In spite of physical limitations, you have been given a precious opportunity. You can find out who you are. And you will! I wish you good luck.

Jake, 38 years old, "We each write our own script entitled 'Life Happens.'"
(**Note:** Jake is a screenplay writer and artist. At the time of his back injury, he was the personal aide to a major motion picture director. His story was sent to me in the following screenplay form.)

FADE IN

INTERIORS-BEAKINS STORAGE-DAY

Our hero, Jake, is schlepping boxes of sound-track tape for the esteemed director at his studio (the envy and wonder of the civilized world, home of proven hits). He seems a lost soul, consigned to an existential hell of endless, dimly lit wooden corridors. Using his best straight-back, tight-gut, bent-knee technique, he lifts a fatal box of sound-effects reels. Jake's expression suddenly changes as he feels his lower back muscles give way with a sound effect for an audience of one—sheet of plastic tearing.

CUT TO ONE YEAR LATER

INTERIORS-JAKE'S BEDROOM, ST. HELENA, CALIFORNIA-DAY

Lucky for Jake, he's married to a loving wife and has a thirteen-year-old daughter, because at this point there's not much he enjoys or can do for himself. He spends his time trying not to move, cough, or even breathe too hard because all of that sends his lower back into spasms—thirty-second torture zones where he is transfixed by an invisible railroad spike rammed right into L5S1. Lying on one's back hour after hour, one's lungs fill with fluid, and eventually one is forced to cough and suffer the consequences.

Part of his depression is that although he is thirty-one-years old, Jake feels about a hundred. He looks totally defeated. The ten-foot walk to the bathroom is a big deal. He cannot find comfort anywhere; even his underwear is a struggle, as it is not designed for blown disks. Nor are his shoes and socks. He can't walk or drive anywhere. All of his musculature is slowly melting away. Jake feels and looks frustrated and angry.

Three doctors have recommended surgery—"We can get you on the table next Tuesday." But Jake, your humble narrator, has the sneaking suspicion he can beat the rap without getting sliced and diced.

JAKE SPEAKING:

The body is tricky, be good to it! I had a ninety-nine percent perfectly healthy male body that was rendered inert due to the one percent that strained. I am afraid. How bad was this going to get? Would I recover and be able to function and if so, to what degree? I must get better without surgery, on my own and with the help of bodyworkers.

JAKE SPEAKING TWO YEARS LATER, no longer working in film:

My situation would have been very difficult without my family around to help. Just their presence and concern made me feel courageous and hopeful, even after two years of pain and disability. Oddly enough, the fact that my wife and daughter made constant fun of me, my crab walk, the amount of time it took to do anything, etc., helped me a lot! Being able to see the comic and absurd side of the situation kept me from taking myself too seriously.

One night I was alone in the house, as Marta and Mia had gone shopping. I was lying on my back in bed, knees up on two pillows. It was winter, and I was wearing a warm sweater. Marta had turned on the heat before she left and now the sweater was too hot. I carefully and slowly tried to sneak the sweater off without my back knowing. An hour later, after numerous spasms, I was totally worn out. I had only been able to maneuver my sweater over my head, so now my head was stuck in the sweater. I burst into tears of rage and frustration, and that's how my family found me, crying with my head in the sweater.

Pain is physically and spiritually exhausting. I finally found my way out of pain through physical exercise: swimming, yoga, and riding a bike! I channeled my anger toward healing. I used this energy to be willful against an enemy, pain. I used my quieter energy for healing meditation and visualization. With this, in addition to the love and support of my family, I moved successfully beyond unwanted disability.

Martha, 47 years old, "Bed rest bliss!"

At the time I was bedridden, I was working twenty hours per week. My employer was very supportive of my pregnancy with triplets. He let me use sick leave and maternity leave.

My husband worked long hours, but when he was home, he was very attentive. It also helped that his parents visited twice a week and brought dinner. We had student tenants living in our home, and the three males were somewhat helpful. It was nice to know they were there in case of an emergency. We hired a female grad student to cook for us and help with housecleaning.

I was a happy beached whale. My favorite meal was fresh-squeezed orange juice with Metamucil for breakfast. I usually ate a snack of apples and cheese, a sandwich for lunch, and a normal dinner with everyone. I had an appetite like an elephant, but I looked more like a whale. Every day, I made sure to have four meat and dairy servings, lots of fruit, nothing fried, spicy, or sweet, and a lot of milk.

I had little trouble tolerating bed rest. Once the kitchen butcher block with four wheels was converted to a trolley cart, I was organized and well stocked to spend hours by myself. This is where we kept the essentials: a gallon jug of water, books and my journal, my lunch and snacks, the phone. My ob-gyn actually came to our home twice a week, and so did a masseuse! The hours sailed slowly by but I enjoyed the time, listening to Indian ragas, drinking my gallons of water, and watching films. I know others who were bedridden and fought it. When I learned I had to be bedridden, I cried, and then committed myself to keeping things simple and finding peace.

My husband looks back on it and always describes me as "in the zone." I called it "incubator bliss." I was content lying down; I'm not really sure how long I would have been able to stand. I was enormous, and growing larger every day. The two hours that I spent each day sitting up in our cooled-down hot tub was good for me; it provided new scenery and supported a somewhat challenging time with digestion. The hot tub (cool, not hot) was the brilliant suggestion of a neighbor, and it turned out to be very positive.

In some sense, I felt like I was temporarily on vacation from life's normal responsibilities. All I had to do was grow those little babies inside of me. I was very happy.

CHAPTER TEN

AFFECTION, SEXUALITY, AND BED REST

The uncompromising reality of immobility can be *equally challenging* for patient and loved ones, yet *no one* has to experience alienation or isolation. Rather, it can be a time to marvel, reprioritize, and focus on what you *have,* and what you are *able* to do throughout recovery. With an open heart and positive mind-set, there are endless ways to make the most of this situation, including sharing love and expressing special feelings at all levels.

Let's start with warmth and affection. There are countless ways to fulfill the indisputable need and desire for affection. Similarly, there are plenty of opportunities to enjoy pleasures of love and sexual intimacy. Patience is paramount in the midst of these extenuating circumstances while the desire for *connection* is more important than ever due to medically imposed limitations. With insight to a new emotional and physical landscape, this aspect of recovery can continue in a healthy and wonderful way!

The basics: All human beings thrive best with attention and care. Exhaustive research shows that injury and illness elicit stronger desires for physical and emotional contact in most cases. When a medical ailment causes physical confinement, opportunities to interact are altered or reduced, irrespective of the desires. Yet being confined due to injury or recovery in bed or wheelchair, or from two broken arms, or having to stay hospitalized without privacy, is cause for connecting in boundless ways, from the beginning to the end of the predicament!

Beyond the basics: Sex and immobility might sound like an oxymoron. Think again. A loved one who is confined is the target of much desire. Caring between loved ones at a time like this is compelling! Feelings of isolation, fear, and frustration elicit a special sensation: the urgency to love and to be loved. No one need misunderstand or shut this down!

When physical restriction exists between sexually active people, intimacy commands new, alternative, and creative ways of feeling, giving, and communicating. Medications, physical limitations, erectile dysfunction and/or reduced sensation, and in some cases, catheters (external or indwelling), are common interferences with typical intercourse. Fortunately, the whole body is covered with sensitive receptor cells capable of being pleasured in an infinite variety of ways. Subsequently, it's completely possible for affection and sex to continue when you use your imagination.

Partners who become more aware of each other, with or without immobility conditions, constantly redefine pleasure and the joys of active sex. Lovemaking indeed takes time, but it doesn't always require a full morning or evening, just the quality moments to feel, listen, and learn from each other.

When Hannah Kaiser broke both arms while running in her neighborhood, she was initially "devastated" by the sudden limitations forced upon her. She could not wash or feed herself, wipe herself on the toilet, bathe, brush or floss teeth, or insert tampons. Her husband did *everything* for four weeks while a wrist-to-shoulder cast set each arm. Hannah soon found "humor, grace, and direction" from the accident, and consciously discarded feeling "exposed, fragile, and weak." She learned new ways to function independently, by using her chin, knees, and forehead. She and her husband laughed and cried together, and soon discovered a magical world of sexual exploration. All new seduction presented all new positions and sensations. Hannah shared that while disabled, she lost her fragility. Together, they made the most of Hannah's injury, and treasured their wildly unexpected life adventure!

Peter Stock broke both heels when he fell off a ladder painting his newly purchased home. As a young, hard-working man, he continued working wearing two fracture boots—he wanted this home perfect for his new bride. He painted rooms and polished floors, until he slipped on the sparkling stairs, breaking his left tibia just above the left fracture boot. He and his bride fell even more deeply in love while he spent the next seven weeks in a wheelchair. Julie cooked and cared for him, and sat on his lap to feed him, hug him, love him.

While I was seven months pregnant and bedridden with preterm labor, my husband's gentle words and strokes of affection meant more to me than anything else. Over the weeks as I tripled in size with our first child, we found new ways to be close while loving *very* gently (or the contractions would begin!). I later learned that even the lightest gestures of affection helped my husband deeply; he needed me as much as I needed him. For three months of lying in bed intensely still, our hearts did a lot of dancing! The bed rest experience can offer all relationships an extraordinary connection that might not otherwise occur.

Basic Ways to Improve Intimacy

For encouraging and creating open and loving relationships, warm up the heart with two questions as a mental affirmation or entry in a journal:

What do I think would help make others in my life feel good?

What would help me to feel good right now?

Gentle Displays of Affection

Listening: a simple act that greatly improves trust and communication. It may not always be the bedridden person who needs the ear.

Breathing together: breathing deeply influences our state of mind, and when shared between people, it elicits vitality and joy. Breathing deeply produces new energy and power, and for all human beings, enriches body, mind, and spirit. Like anything else when shared, a new level of energy, warmth, and understanding emerges between two people or a group of friends. When my contractions flared up at night, my husband would calm me by lying close and guiding me in breathing. We would breathe together for as long as it took to feel calm and ensure the contractions ceased. Hints: Exhaling more slowly than inhaling calms the mind. Inhaling more slowly than exhaling energizes it. Balancing the two breaths calms the whole body.

Exchanging love poems, notes of appreciation, drawings, simple gifts: Every Sunday afternoon, my two-year-old niece came to visit. She insisted on getting into bed with me, shoes on, too. She had a gift each time and it was just between the two of us, she didn't want anyone else to see. Way under the sheets, she provided her colorful drawing. We each felt especially loved; it was our special *intimate* time. Emily, now twenty-five years old, is especially close to me. She inspired me while I was bedridden both times, to start every week with notes of gratitude for special people: family, neighbors, and work associates.

Enhancing Intimacy
Verbal affection:
Words of encouragement, appreciation, validation
Questions displaying genuine interest
Physical affection:
Kisses, hugs, smiles, laughter
Massage—helps fight depression and hypertension
Cuddling and sleeping skin-to-skin—it is loving, lowers blood pressure, strengthens the immune system. Skin is considered to be the largest sex organ and there is great power in soft, gentle touching.
Holding hands, wrapping an arm around a shoulder
Rubbing necks, arms, shoulders, head, hands, feet
Brushing long hair

While I was pregnant and bedridden, a friend asked to brush my hair during her visit. She brushed and we talked for two hours! A work associate came to visit and held my hand the minute she saw me. Soon I realized she was doing acupressure on each hand, wrist, and arm. Another friend, a professional masseuse, came to visit once a week. She sat at the end of the bed, lifted the sheets and while talking, she worked on my feet.

For intimate exchanges when intercourse is forbidden, especially for pregnancy bed rest, enjoy close cuddling, long soulful kisses, candlelit dinners, listening to music, and reading to each other. For comprehensive guidance for men and women of all ages and sexual identities, *The Ultimate Guide to Sex and Disability* covers the span of possibilities to create a sex life that works.

The silver lining for sexually active people with physical limitations is the joy of experiencing new ways to share, care, and love. When the initial shock from either the medical condition and/or the recovery requirement dissipates, which it does, romantic feelings surface like exposed nerves. Partners' compassion quotients increase, and the capacity to care and cooperate expand. Often, platonic feelings shift between friends, and sexual interests emerge. Distinctly exciting forms of communication develop for bed rest patients and lovers, especially when alternative ways of making love are explored.

Recommended Resources:

The Ultimate Guide to Sex and Disability, by Miriam Kaufman, M.D., Cory Silverberg, and Fran Odette (Cleis Press: San Francisco, 2007).

Enabling Romance, by Ken Kroll and Erica Levy Klein (Harmony Books: New York, 1992).

Sexualhealth.com

POSITIVE AFFIRMATIONS AND HABITS

An affirmation is a positive thought held with conviction to produce a desired result. The use of affirmations is powerful, a tool for shifting consciousness and bringing greater peace into life. I highly recommend finding one affirmation while enduring the time you are physically confined. In both of my bed rest experiences, I used two or three select affirmations. Each was a source of strength and reinforcement, as well as hope, peace, and direction. Today, I use affirmations for almost every aspect of my life, in my athletic and professional pursuits, and for grace in personal matters.

Affirmation(s) can be self-created, and repeated endlessly. The use of a prayer, a poem, a quote, or some other specific declaration can easily be used as well. Write it, email it, print it, post it, and verbally state this positive thought every day. Whatever affirmation(s) you choose, expect results!

I recommend verbalizing your affirmations and repeating them quietly inside your mind. When alone, you can speak the words out loud. If you are visual, look at it and imprint it in your heart. As you say your affirmation, feel it, visualize it, and believe it. It then goes cellular.

There are several affirmations below. If one in particular speaks to you, highlight it, copy it into your phone or laptop, paste it wherever you'll see it and read it. Or, create your own affirmation(s). Read your selection(s) over and over, every day, multiple times per day. When you give this exercise a chance, you will notice an improvement in your energy and spirit. Affirmations reinforce important values. Open your mind and allow these affirmations to guide you to the limitless opportunities made available by your bed rest experience.

I am living every moment to the fullest, on or off bed rest.

I am here to learn.

I am true to myself, always, and I accept myself as I am.

I shall not agonize over this problem. I choose to greet life with courage, joy, and good humor.

I am self-sufficient, especially with the right tools, a good attitude, and determination.

I respect the patterns and fluctuations of my unique life, feeling empowered wherever I am.

I am capable of making a positive difference all around me, even when I am bedridden.

I acknowledge my physical weakness, and I feel strong.

I am flexible, resourceful, and open to new possibilities. I can adjust to life's changes, and I feel no need to resist. What is, is what is now.

I will bend and grow, adjusting to the winds of change. Bed rest is an opportunity for me, right now.

I am invigorated when I look at my life and know that I can accept bed rest and work with it.

Life has many options. I am creative and resourceful.

I can help myself and others so no one is lost.

I will use all resources wisely so nothing is wasted.

I take many deep breaths and practice nonresistance.

I take many deep breaths and practice patience.

I live with courage and compassion.

I have a reverence for life, and a faith in the larger process. This faith sustains my experience, on or off bed rest. This faith affirms who I need to be at any moment. This faith affirms that I am on bed rest, and I will make the best of it.

I respect and embrace nature. In nature, everything is valuable; everything has its place. A rose, a daisy, a lark, a squirrel each manifests its potential differently, and beautifully. On bed rest, I am still like a rock set on a hill. Like the rock, I move very little. I participate from my own place in life. The rock does not suffer from low self-esteem, nor do I.

Every day of bed rest is one in a succession of special days where I am creating an experience that allows me to prosper.

To make bed rest a meaningful existence, I am conscious of balancing giving and receiving.

The Serenity Prayer by theologian Reinhold Niebuhr:

God, grant me the serenity to accept the things I cannot change,

Courage to change the things I can,

And the wisdom to know the difference.

Positive Habits for Making the Most of Bed Rest

Be optimistic.

Focus on the positive.

Perform acts of kindness; it releases serotonin in your brain. (Serotonin is a substance that has tremendous health benefits.)

Wear clean clothes.

Have fun, laugh!

Express gratitude.

Smile at helpers, visitors, your food, your utensils, your hands.

Nurture what is important to you.

Take care of your body.

Accomplish what you can with the resources you have.

Use your imagination.

Seek humor.

Create something to perpetuate what you love to see, smell,
    taste, and hear.

Create an event to look forward to.

Be inspired.

Breathe deeply.

Be organized.

Eat well; stay hydrated.

Write fresh goals for every day.

Help others in any way that's possible.

Share your expertise.

Repeat affirmations for personal reinforcement.

Completely engage in your experience(s).

Savor happy moments.

Avoid negativity, including negative people.

The Author's Own Life Credo:

Seek wisdom from Nature.

Live in truth.

Give more than you take.

Love deeply.

Say thank you.

Begin again.

PERSONAL CALENDAR AND JOURNAL

Date:_____ Day of Week: _____

Goals for the Day: _____

	APPOINTMENTS	MEDICINE MANAGEMENT	EXERCISE	OTHER
5:00 a.m.				
6:00 a.m.				
7:00 a.m.				
8:00 a.m.				
9:00 a.m.				
10:00 a.m.				
11:00 a.m.				
12:00 p.m.				
1:00 p.m.				
2:00 p.m.				
3:00 p.m.				
4:00 p.m.				
5:00 p.m.				
6:00 p.m.				
7:00 p.m.				
8:00 p.m.				
9:00 p.m.				
10:00 p.m.				
11:00 p.m.				
12:00 a.m.				

Mindful Notes: _____

_____

Use the personal calendar on page 131 to organize your life while on bed rest. Keeping close track of the events of your days provides structure and purpose to your new personal regime and is extremely therapeutic.

Make room in your day to journal and follow your thoughts during this introspective time. The page below is a model for you, but journal in a format that works for you: write in a blank journal, type in a Word document, or artistically hand-letter entries on craft paper.

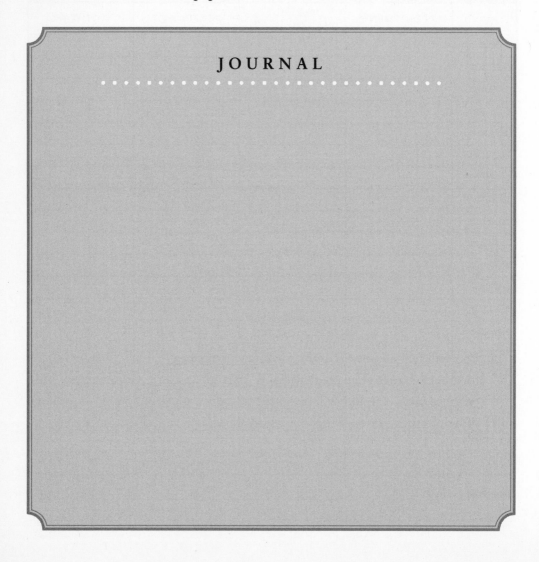

JOURNAL

MEDICAL TEAM

When any unexpected and serious medical situation occurs, it is imperative to stay in close contact with your medical team and to be organized about the many aspects of your care. Frequently, if patients or caregivers don't initiate contact, there will be little to none. Take advantage of your resources, and optimize the medical expertise for information and excellent advice en route to a successful recovery.

This organizer encourages you to list your medical team, log your questions, and track your answers. There may be difficulty in thinking clearly, remembering to ask the right questions, and listening while at the same time understanding the answers.

1. It is your right to request time with your doctor and medical team. A planned telephone appointment will provide proper focus for every question and thorough medical explanations.
2. Approach your physician with respect and demand the same in return.
3. Prepare your concerns before your conversations and ask all questions in a direct but non-threatening way.
4. Be specific when describing symptoms and the circumstances around any medical changes. Only you know exactly how you feel, where, when, etc.
5. You will feel empowered when you and your health-care providers work together to treat your medical issue. This kind of approach will not only enhance your care but will also help to reduce stress and alleviate feelings of helplessness, hopelessness, incompetence, anger, and fear.

Who's Who at the Doctor's Office

1. *Physician*

Name _____

Phone Number _____

Email address _____

_____

Office Emergency Phone Number _____

Hospital Phone Number _____

Doctor's Home Number (if appropriate) _____

Date—Question/Answer: _____

_____

_____

_____

Date—Question/Answer: _____

_____

_____

_____

Date—Question/Answer: _____

_____

_____

_____

Date—Question/Answer: _____

_____

_____

Important points my doctor has emphasized for optimal recovery: _____

_____

_____

_____

_____

2. Back-up Physician: Partners, On-call Backup Team, etc.

Name _____

Phone Number _____

Email address _____

Office Emergency Phone Number _____

Name _____

Phone Number _____

Email address _____

Office Emergency Phone Number _____

3. Other Medical Staff: Nurses, Physical Therapists, etc.

Name _____

Phone Number _____

Email address _____

This person's unique role in my recovery: _____

Name _____

Phone Number _____

Email address _____

This person's unique role in my recovery: _____

Name _____

Phone Number _____

Email address _____

This person's unique role in my recovery: _____

4. Other Professionals: Bodyworkers, Lab Technicians, Pain Management People, Pharmacists, etc.

Name _____

Phone Number _____

Email address _____

_____

This person's unique role in my recovery: _____

_____

_____

_____

Name _____

Phone Number _____

Email address _____

_____

This person's unique role in my recovery: _____

_____

_____

_____

Name _____

Phone Number _____

Email address _____

_____

This person's unique role in my recovery: _____

_____

_____

_____

APPENDIX D

POSTCARDS FROM THE BED

Here are some sample postcards. Copy these or create your own. "Send" to the cook in the kitchen, to a neighbor who just helped you, or to anyone you feel like writing!

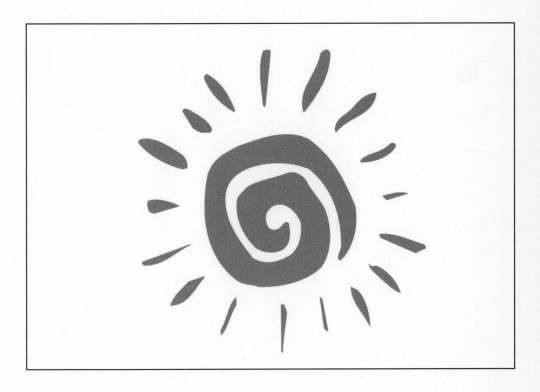

To:

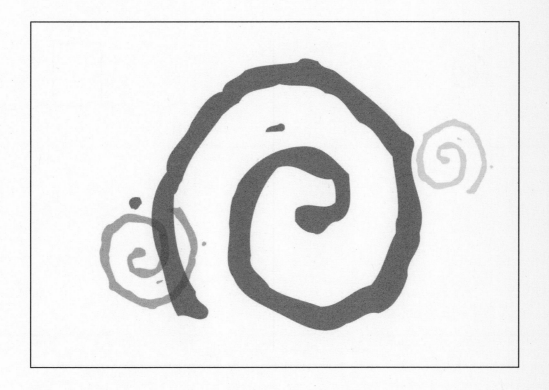

To:

NEW CONTACTS AND RESOURCES

Name:_____

Email:_____

Telephone:_____

Address:_____

City, State, Zip:_____

Notes:_____

_____

_____

Name:_____

Email:_____

Telephone:_____

Address:_____

City, State, Zip:_____

Notes:_____

_____

_____

Name:_____

Email:_____

Telephone:_____

Address:_____

City, State, Zip:_____

Notes:_____

_____

_____

Name:_____

Email:_____

Telephone:_____

Address:_____

City, State, Zip:_____

Notes:_____

_____

_____

_____

Name:_____

Email:_____

Telephone:_____

Address:_____

City, State, Zip:_____

Notes:_____

_____

_____

_____

Name:_____

Email:_____

Telephone:_____

Address:_____

City, State, Zip:_____

Notes:_____

_____

_____

_____

APPENDIX F

SHOPPING GUIDE

Shopping is most successfully accomplished over the Internet. There are endless resources for groceries, pharmaceutical supplies, clothing, bedding, pet supplies, electronics, cosmetics, and cleansers. Just search online for whatever you are looking for. Your online shopping adventure will begin! For a mail order catalog, I advise calling the toll-free phone number for each individual catalog, and requesting that your name be put on the mailing list. Or try www.catalogs.com for a comprehensive selection of mail order catalogs by category.

If television is your preferred medium, there are a number of cable stations dedicated to shopping.

My Favorite and Most Helpful Catalogs

L.L. Bean 800.514.2326 www.llbean.com (clothes, lightweight cots, camping)

The Company Store 800.285.3696 www.thecompanystore.com (pillows, mattresses, sheets, towels)

Williams Sonoma 800.541.2233 www.williams-sonoma.com (kitchen, appliances)

Chambers Bedding 800.334.9790 www.wshome.com (robes, sheets, etc.)

Pottery Barn 888.779.5176 www.potterybarn.com (furniture, bedding, rugs, outdoor)

The Container Store 888.contain (888.266.8246) www.thecontainerstore.com (containers, cleaning, organizers, accessories)

For Children and Baby's Clothing (including maternity for mothers), Baby Basics, Books, Toys, Safety, and Educational Supplies

Hearth Song 800.533.4397 www.hearthsong.com

Hannah Anderson 800.222.0544 www.hannahanderson.com (clothes, accessories)

Biobottoms at Diaper Junction 877.791.8065 www.diaperjunction.com
Diapers and More 800.342.7377 www.diapers.com
One Step Ahead 800.274.8440 www.onestepahead.com (all baby care)
ChildCraft 800.631.5652 www.childcraft.com (educational products)
Sensational Beginnings 800.444.2147 www.sensationalbeginnings.com

For Health Care and Home Care Supply Catalogs

Bed Bath and Beyond 800.462.3966 www.bedbathandbeyond.com
BackSaver 800.748.9376 www.backsaver.com (furniture and accessories)
Gaiam Living Arts 877.989.6321 www.gaiam.com (household, health care)
Levenger 800.544.0880 www.levenger.com (able table, over-bed tables, etc.)
The Container Store 888.contain (888.266.8246) www.thecontainerstore.
   com (containers, cleaning, organizers, accessories)
Hands-On Health Care Catalog 800.442.2232—The Acupressure Institute

For Magazine Subscriptions

Audubon 212.979.3000
Better Homes & Garden 800.374.4244
Black Enterprise 800.727.7777
Business Week 800.635.1200
Ebony 800.999.5954
The Economist 800.456.6086
Elle 800.876.8775
Entertainment Weekly 800.541.1000
Family Life 707.586.9562
Financial Times 800.628.8088
Forbes 800.888.9896
Fortune 800.541.1000
Gourmet 800.888.8728
Harper's 800.444.4653
InStyle 800.274.6200
Inc. 800.234.0999

International Herald Tribune 800.882.2884
Internet World 800.573.3062
Investor's Business Daily 800.831.2525
Ladies' Home Journal 800.374.4545
Mac Home Journal 800.800.6542
Money Magazine 800.541.1000
National Geographic 800.NGS.LINE
Nation's Business 800.873.4769
New Republic 800.827.1289
New Yorker 800.825.2510
New York Times 800.631.2500
Newsweek 800.631.1040
Outside 800.678.1131
PC Magazine 800.335.1195
PC Today 800.544.1296
PC World 800.825.7595
People 800.541.1000
Ranger Rick 800.588.1650
Reader's Digest 800.234.9000
Road & Track 800.876.8316
Scientific America 800.333.1199
Ski 800.238.1616
Sports Illustrated 800.541.1000
Time 800.541.1000
Travel & Leisure 800.888.8728
USA Today 800.USA.0001
U.S. News & World Report 800.544.9224
Vogue 800.234.2347
The Wall Street Journal 800.345.8502
Working Mother 800.627.0690
Working Woman 800.234.9675
Worth 800.777.1851

ABOUT THE AUTHOR

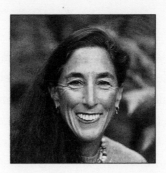

BARBARA EDELSTON PETERSON has dedicated her life to health and wellness, and improving the lives of people of all ages through exercise, self-awareness, and the power of positive thinking. Now fifty-six years old, she is an author, motivational speaker, sports psychologist, world-class triathlete, wife, and mother of two daughters. She is uniquely qualified to inspire and educate people recovering from physical limitations as a result of injury, illness, or pregnancy. Barbara is the author of *The Bed Rest Survival Guide* (1998), the founder of The Power of Exercise, and is a contributor to *Ms. Fitness*, *Triathlete*, and *Women's Health*. To contact Barbara and to read her blog, please visit her website at www.bedrestwellness.com. She lives in Berkeley, California.

Photograph by Joan Lakin Mikkelsen.

TO OUR READERS

Viva Editions publishes books that inform, enlighten, and entertain. We do our best to bring you, the reader, quality books that celebrate life, inspire the mind, revive the spirit, and enhance lives all around. Our authors are practical visionaries: people who offer deep wisdom in a hopeful and helpful manner. Viva was launched with an attitude of growth and we want to spread our joy and offer our support and advice where we can to help you live the Viva way: vivaciously!

We're grateful for all our readers and want to keep bringing you books for inspired living. We invite you to write to us with your comments and suggestions, and what you'd like to see more of. You can also sign up for our online newsletter to learn about new titles, author events, and special offers.

Viva Editions
2246 Sixth St.
Berkeley, CA 94710
www.vivaeditions.com
(800) 780-2279
Follow us on Twitter @vivaeditions
Friend/fan us on Facebook